Look after your Back

Note: The techniques and applications described in this book were examined and approved by experts. The instructions are for the use of physically and mentally healthy people. If you are receiving medical care, or if you feel ill, please consult your doctor as to whether the procedures described and the techniques demonstrated are suitable for you. People are not all alike. If you experience any pain or other problems while using these procedures, whether once or several times, discontinue the procedures. Neither the author nor the publisher can take responsibility for possible damage or injury which might occur in connection with following the instructions contained in this book.

Copyright © 1998 Könemann Verlagsgesellschaft mbH
Bonner Str. 126, D-50968 Cologne

Realization: Könemann Verlagsgesellschaft mbH
Editor: KVM Dr. Kolster und Co. Produktions- und
Verlags-GmbH, Marburg
Photography: Lutz Pape
Editor: Dr. Sabine Klapp
Layout: LOGO
Graphic Design: Gabriela Bauer, L. Lamm (p.13), Authors (p.22/23)
Cover Design: Peter Feierabend, Steffi Weischer

Original title: Gutes für jeden Rücken

Copyright © 1999 for the English edition
Könemann Verlagsgesellschaft mbH

Translation from German: Phil Greenhead
Editor of the English-language Edition: Lynn Brown in association with
Goodfellow & Egan, Cambridge
Typesetting: Goodfellow and Egan, Cambridge
Project Manager for Goodfellow & Egan: Jackie Dobbyne
Managing Editor: Bettina Kaufmann
Project Management: Kristin Zeier
Production Manager: Detlev Schaper
Assistants: Nicola Leurs, Alexandra Kiesling
Printing and Binding: Sing Cheong Printing Co. Ltd., Hong Kong

Printed in Hong Kong, China

ISBN 3-8290-2008-2

10 9 8 7 6 5 4 3 2 1

Look after your Back

Dr. Bernard Kolster
Astrid Frank

Recently Developed Exercise Programs

Avoid incorrect posture
Exercises for every day

KÖNEMANN

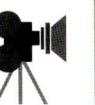

Summary of video contents

Method	Minutes into tape
Posture training	.1:35
Getting up	.1:50
Sitting	.2:05
Standing	.2:45
Lifting, bending, carrying	.3:20
Lying down	.4:15
Stretching postures	.6:00
Stretching Exercises: Top Ten	.7:25
1. Leg and foot muscles	.7:40
2. Inner thigh muscles	.8:05
3. Hip muscles	.8:40
4. Buttock muscles	.9:10
5. Rear thigh muscles	.9:45
6. Lateral neck muscles	.10:10
7. Rear neck muscles	.10:35
8. Chest and shoulder muscles	.11:10
9. Abdominal muscles	.11:55
10. Finger and hand muscles	.12:20
Strengthening Program 1: Beginners	.12:40
1. Back muscles	.12:55
2. Lateral trunk and hip muscles	.14:30
3. Abdominal muscles	.14:55
Strengthening Program 2: Intermediate	.15:50
1. Back muscles	.16:05
2. Lateral trunk and hip muscles	.17:20
3. Abdominal muscles	.17:55
Strengthening Program 3: Intermediate	.18:55
1. Back muscles	.19:05
2. Lateral trunk and hip muscles	.20:15
3. Abdominal muscles	.20:45

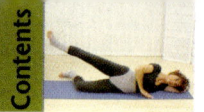

Foreword
Back pain: one symptom … many causes   4

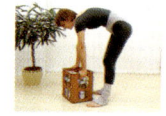

I. Theory: What you should know about your back   7

The structure of your back   7
The spinal column: the framework   7
The intervertebral disks: the pressure cushion   9
The muscles: the motor   11

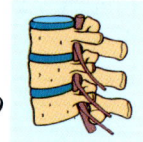

Posture   12
Upright posture and slouching   13
The effects of posture on health   15

Common causes of back pain   20
Bad posture   21
Back strain/stiffness   26
Upper back syndrome   28
Lumbago   30
Damaged vertebra   31
Damaged joints   32
Slipped disk   32
Osteoporosis   34
Diseases of the internal organs   36
Psychosomatic back pain   36

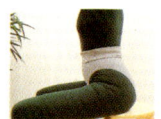

II. Practice: How to keep your back fit   39

Posture training   39
Getting up and lying down   39
Sitting down   40
Standing and walking   44
Bending, lifting and carrying   45
Lying down and sleeping   50
Everyday and work environment   53

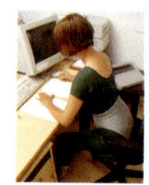

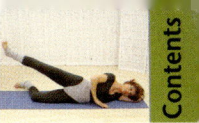

Stretching exercises   55
Stretching postures   55
Top ten stretching exercises for the whole body   57

Strengthening exercises   64
Program 1: Beginners   65
Program 2: Intermediate   69
Program 3: Advanced   72

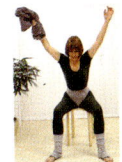

Activities that are kind to the back   76
Walking and hiking   76
Jogging   77
Swimming   78
Cycling   78
Riding   79
Dancing   80

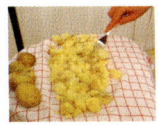

Relaxation and relief for the back   80
Relaxation   80
Relief postures   81
Ways to relieve stress   84
Home heat-treatment remedies   85

Appendix   89

Further reading   89
Index   90

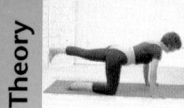

Foreword

Back pain: one symptom ... many causes

Over the years, back problems have become the "people's disease." Almost every individual has suffered from back pain at least once in their life. Back pain itself is the result of a combination of pains and problems, but one thing is certain: whether the pain is in the nape of the neck, between the shoulder blades or in the sacrum, whether it stings, aches or radiates, is stabbing or chronic, anyone who has suffered from it knows how seriously a bad back can affect their well-being.

The fact that there is a whole host of problems is hardly surprising if we bear in mind what complex structures our bodies are. What we generally describe as the back basically consists of many different components: bones, disks, ligaments, muscles and nerves must be in perfect harmony with each other if the back is to "function" without friction. Even a small fault in one of these structures is enough to disturb the balance of the whole. Possible causes of back problems are therefore just as numerous as the symptoms.

Basically, the main causes of problems are changes in the bones, damage to the disks and injuries to the muscles or nerves. However, it is muscle injury that is most often responsible for back problems. Fortunately, it is also the most easily treated – that's why the problems caused by muscles, and the treatment of these, are the focus of this book.

Muscles provide a connection between every section of the body: each routine movement calls on a large number of them to be active throughout the body. Some of them have to contract and hold while others can relax at the same time. This cooperation is perfectly synchronized, time after time, with each movement. Postures and everyday movements that are one-sided disturb and alter this synchronization. The problems

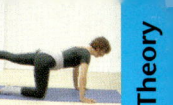

that arise as a result of this, affect the work of the back and may manifest themselves as back pain.

Because of this, muscle-based back pain is not always necessarily based around the backbone; it may be caused by disturbances to the coordination of the muscles in other parts of the body. This is why all the exercises described here include the whole body, from head to toe. When targeting individual muscle groups and their problems, we do of course stress certain points, but basically all the muscles work together, just as they do in normal everyday movement. The likelihood of having a positive effect on back pain is greatly increased when the pain is muscle based; this is when we can all work for ourselves and take action against the pain. Although a complete turnaround is almost impossible once the bones have been damaged by chronic bad posture or disease, the situation can be prevented from deteriora-ting further if the load on the back is correctly distributed on a day-to-day basis. This book will show you how to structure your everyday environ-ment, your posture, and your movements so as to protect your back and keep it healthy.

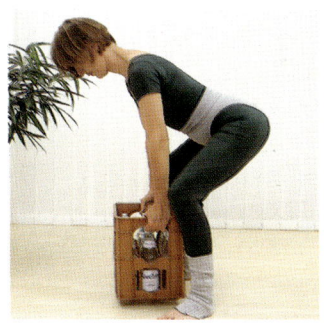

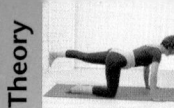

How to use the book and video together

The contents of the book and the video match each other exactly. We recommend that you use them together to get the most from them. The best approach is probably to read the background information on the themes that interest you first; the first section, "Theory", deals with these. After this, take time out to watch the video. This will give you a very good picture of the exercises described in the practical section. If, when you are reading the practical section, you feel the need to watch the more difficult exercises again on video, the camera icon next to the individual exercises will help you to do so. The video running time (in minutes) is given next to these icons. You can easily find the sequence you are looking for by using the minute-counter on your video recorder. Simply set the counter to zero (display in minutes) when you insert the tape and fast-forward to the figure given beside the camera icon.

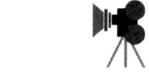

Camera icon

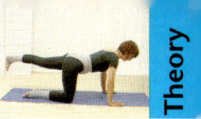

I. Theory: What you should know about your back

The structure of the back

There is a wide variety of causes for undue strain on the back. However, we only generally become aware of it when we feel pain. Pain should be viewed as the body's signal that something is wrong.

To understand how and why we get back pain, it is important to know which elements are involved in back function and how these can be damaged. The three most important of the back's "building blocks" are the vertebral column, the disks and the muscles.

The spinal column: the framework

Together with the ribcage, the vertebral column forms a stable but mobile framework for the trunk. Because it is divided into small segments – the vertebrae – it achieves both optimum mobility and great stability at the same time. Since the segments form a sort of "supply chain," the individual vertebrae are connected to and simultaneously protected from each other by articulations, flexible pads, muscles, tendons, and ligaments.

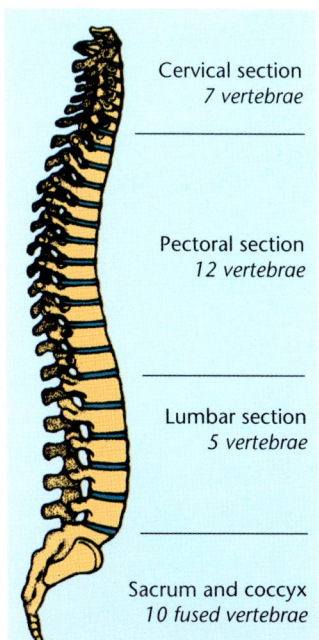

Cervical section
7 vertebrae

Pectoral section
12 vertebrae

Lumbar section
5 vertebrae

Sacrum and coccyx
10 fused vertebrae

The sections of the vertebral column

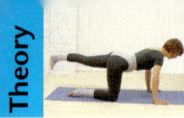
The possibilities for movement created in this manner are controlled by innumerable nerves. The mobile section of the vertebral column, with a total of 24 vertebrae, is divided to correspond with the different sections of the trunk, the cervical, chest, and lumbar regions. Below these we have the sacrum and the coccyx, which together consist of another ten vertebrae.

The ribcage: protection for the lungs and the heart

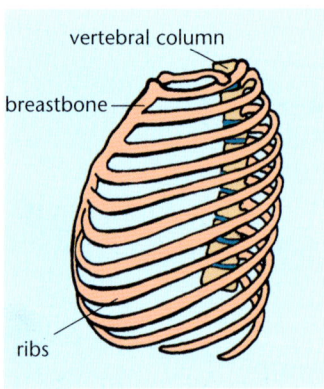

vertebral column

breastbone

ribs

The cervical section of the spine consists of seven vertebrae and is the most mobile section of the vertebral column.

The 12 vertebrae of the chest section connect with the ribs. Together with the breastbone, they form the ribcage, which protects the lungs and heart. The pectoral girdle rests on the ribcage. Below the pectoral vertebrae are the five vertebrae of the lumbar region. As these have to carry the most weight and are most heavily involved when there are damaging movements, they are particularly thick and sturdy.

Finally, the sacrum and the coccyx form the lower end of the vertebral column. These ten vertebrae are no longer mobile and have fused together. The sacrum and the coccyx, the two iliac bones, the two pubic bones, and the two ischia together form the pelvis.

Each vertebra consists of a compact vertebral body and the vertebral arch with its transverse processes and spinate processes. The two upper cervical vertebrae are an exception to this. They are differently shaped to facilitate the rotational movement of the head.

The vertebral arch surrounds the spinal cord, the most important nerve path between the brain and the body. Between each vertebra the so-called local nerves branch off from the spinal cord. These deliver impulses from the

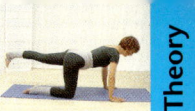

brain to the muscles in the body. In reverse, perceptual information is sent from the body to the brain.

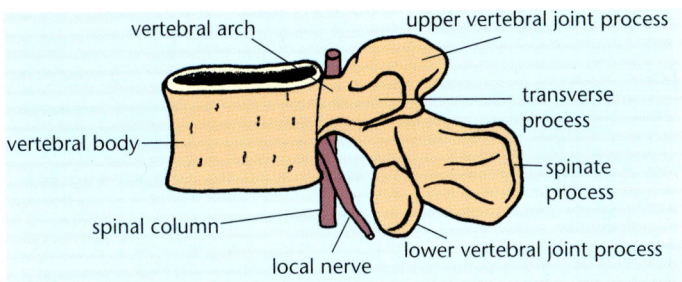

The vertebra: the load-bearing component of the vertebral column

Above and below the two transverse processes of each vertebra are the small vertebral joints. With the intervertebral disks, these provide a flexible connection between the vertebrae and therefore ensure mobility of the vertebral column. In addition, the transverse processes and the spinate processes form attachment points for the muscles. The spinate processes are, moreover, the bony processes we know as the "vertebral column" and we can see and feel these from the outside. The vertebrae themselves are deep inside the body.

The intervertebral disks: the pressure cushion

The disks lie between the individual vertebral bodies. Their task is to act as a buffer between the bony vertebrae. They consist of a flexible fibrous ring and a gelatinous core and they yield to pressure.

If the intervertebral disks did not cushion the "spaces" between the bony vertebrae, we would be able to feel every shock to the body, uncushioned, right into the head. It is only through the cushioning effect of the disks that the impact of, for example, taking a step when walking, is absorbed.

The frequent pressure on the disks during the day means that they gradually give off liquid from the core into their immediate environment. This makes them

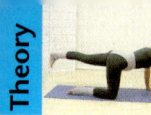

Theory

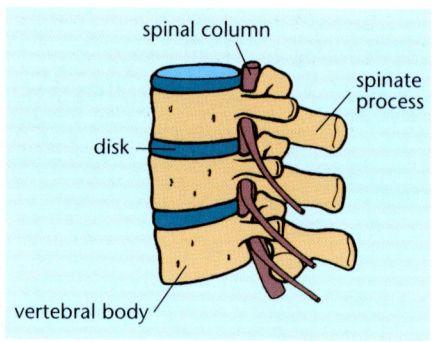

The disks: "shock absorbers" between the vertebrae

spinal column

spinate process

disk

vertebral body

thinner and less flexible. On the other hand, when lying down overnight, the vertebral column is relieved of this pressure. In this position, the disks are able to take up liquid and nutrients from their environment. This is why we are a little taller when we get up in the morning than in the evening after a day in the vertical position. When they are full to bursting the disks are at their most flexible and best able to perform under pressure.

The ability of the disks to alternate between taking up liquid and giving it off deteriorates the more frequently they are put under pressure, something that usually occurs with age. Their flexibility is retained and promoted to best effect by regularly alternating periods of pressure and relaxation.

But even the periods under pressure may have a distinctly different effect on the disks, depending on the pressure distribution. If the vertebral column is stretched out in an upright position, the pressure on the disks is evenly distributed at every point. On the other hand, a hunched, forward-bending body posture means one-

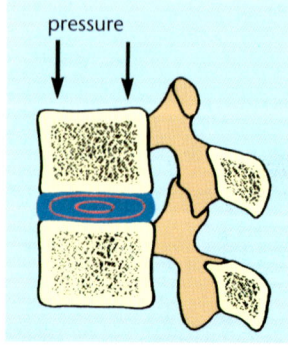

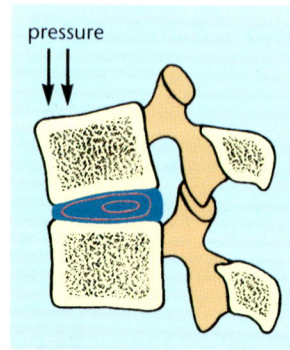

Comparison of equal and asymmetrical pressure on the disks

pressure

pressure

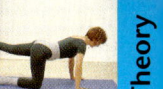

sided pressure on the disks. In the long term this may deform them and the outer side of a disk may tear. Measurements of the pressure on disks in the lower back have shown that the overall pressure is greater when sitting rather than standing. The pressure on the disks also increases considerably when lifting something with a hunched, bent posture.

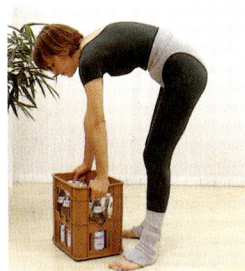

Lifting wrongly: one-sided, increased pressure on the disks

The muscles: the motor

The posture and movement of the human body are dependent on the work of the muscles. But this never means using just one muscle to carry out one movement or hold one posture. Even small, specific movements will require several muscles to work together. Complex coordination of all the muscles in the body is required in order to hold the body upright against the force of gravity.

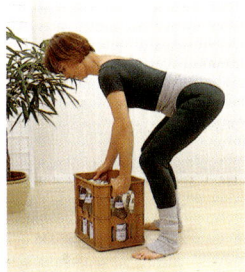

Lifting correctly: evenly distributed, lower pressure on the disks

The back muscles make a major contribution, but not the only one by a long way. Differing in length over each section, they run parallel to the vertebral column, from the neck to the pelvis, and pull the vertebral column up and back. The side and front hold is provided by the stomach muscles, which have

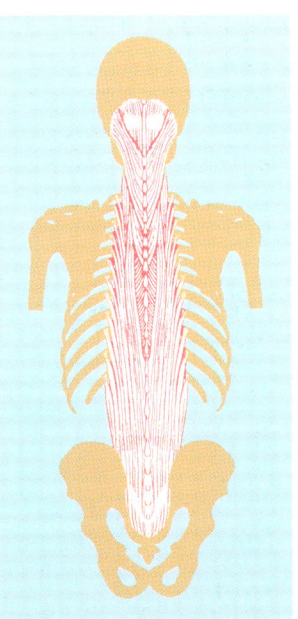

The long back muscles pull the vertebral column back

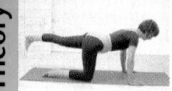
a partial backward effect and which hold the trunk to the sides and in front. The pelvic and leg muscles pull the pelvis into a slightly forward-tilted position and hold the legs upright. The tension of the shoulder and arm muscles holds the pectoral girdle in a central position over the ribcage.

In addition to the muscles, powerful ligaments stabilize the vertebral column, holding the individual vertebrae and disks in place.

Posture

Through the process of evolution, humans have developed from being four-legged to two-legged. We might think the whole "problem" only began when we adopted an upright posture, but this is not so. If we look closely at the anatomy of the human body, we come to the conclusion that it is very well made to cope with being upright on two legs. From close examination and assessment we can see that one decisive element is that all the physical structures should be in the best position and subject to the optimum workload: this is the case with "upright posture." An upright posture is adopted throughout the different stages of development, even in infancy. When lying face down, the internal cavity in the lower back and the cervical vertebrae are supported and, later, when a baby begins to pull itself up, it has to make more of an effort against the force of gravity. If you sit a child up too early, before it can hold itself up, the vertebral column sinks to make a hunched back. This is how bad posture is pre-programmed even at this stage. A sitting position is only suitable for babies when the back muscles are strong enough to hold the trunk upright.

Body posture is learned during infancy

If a child's muscles and posture are to continue to develop healthily later, it is important that they move about a lot from day to day. However, as they get older, the length of time children are expected to sit increases constantly: in nurseries and at school, for instance. If the

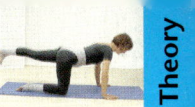

muscles are not stimulated and strengthened by sufficient periods of activity, the muscles holding the trunk tire more quickly and revert to the sunken, "hunched" posture. Unsuitable furniture can encourage this trend if it is not designed with the physical proportions of children in mind. (For more on correct seating, see page 53.)

Upright posture and slouching

The distinction between the "upright" and the "hunched" or "slouching" posture was a result of decades of research work by Dr. Alois Bruegger. The "cog wheel" model he designed provides an excellent comparison of the difference between the hunched and upright posture when sitting.

The cog wheels represent the movement of the vertebral column. The lower cog corresponds to the tipped pelvis, the middle cog demonstrates the lift of the ribcage, and the upper cog shows the extension of the neck.

With the cog wheel model, the link between the different sections of the body are clearly shown: when the lower wheel turns forward and down, the pelvis tips and the ribcage is encouraged to lift forward and upward. As a result, the neck extends slightly and the upright posture is achieved. On the other hand, if the pelvis "rolls" back, the ribcage sinks inward and the cervical vertebrae and chin are pushed outward meaning that the hunched posture prevails.

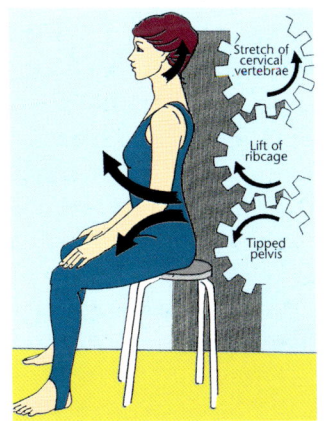

The "cog wheel model" according to Dr. Bruegger, representing the action of the vertebral column

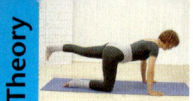

A simple awareness exercise
Take a moment while you are reading this book to imagine that you had frozen at this precise point in time. Now, in your mind, go through your body and feel which way the cogs would be going. Is your pelvis tilted forward or curving back? Is your back hunched or straight and well balanced – the ribcage raised or sunk? Is your neck upright and straight or is your chin sticking forward? Are your shoulders hanging forward or are they to either side? Are both your feet placed firmly on the floor?

In doing this exercise most people would find that they are tending more to the hunched posture than the upright one.

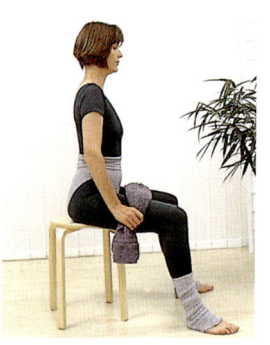

With the upright posture, the vertebral column assumes its natural S-shape

How to achieve an upright posture
With upright posture, the vertebral column adopts its natural elongated S-shape.

This is most easily described in the sitting position:

- the pelvis is tilted slightly forward and downward
- the load is supported by the front section of the ischium
- the ribcage is raised forward and upward
- the lumbar and lower pectoral vertebrae are extended and aligned
- the pectoral girdle is centrally positioned on the ribcage
- the shoulder joints are to either side
- the neck is extended
- the position of the head extends the line of the vertebral column.

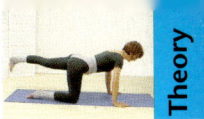

What does the hunched posture look like?

If a hunched posture is adopted, the normal S-curves of the vertebral column are unnaturally affected. The S-shape becomes one long single curve. This is also best described in the sitting position:

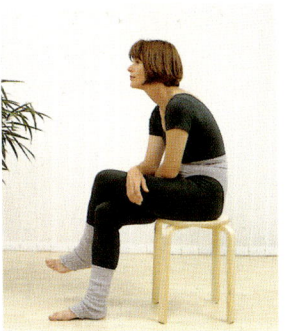

With a hunched posture, the S-shape becomes one long curve

- the pelvis is curved backward and the load is supported at a point behind the ischium
- the ribcage is sunken inward, the pectoral and lumbar vertebrae form a humped back
- the pectoral girdle slips forward over the ribcage
- the shoulder joints are pulled forward
- the head is pushed forward and the cervical vertebrae are excessively over-extended
- there are folds in the neck.

The differences between upright and hunched posture are also apparent when standing and walking. But the differences in the pelvic and lumbar regions are not so clearly obvious as when sitting.

The effects of posture on health

Positive effects of upright posture

With an upright posture, the vertebral column adopts its natural elongated curves. This means that equal pressure is being applied to all the vertebrae because the body of each vertebra and the disks between are all under the same load and are "in play" for longer.

When the vertebral column is in the correct functional position, the body's other joints are also correctly aligned to each other. Their field of movement can therefore be utilized to maximum effect. The disks that stabilize the

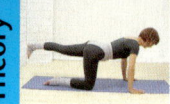

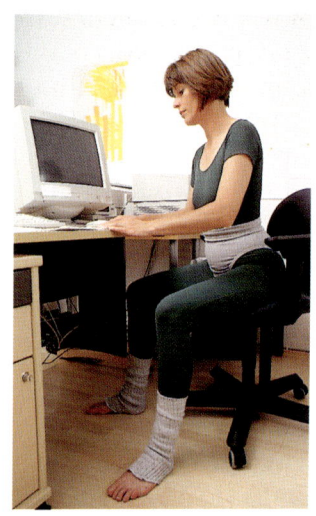

Every physical structure is used to the optimum and evenly loaded

joints achieve their optimum load levels and are not over- or under-exposed to asymmetrical pressure. The same applies to the muscles. When the body is held upright, they are correctly positioned for work and can perform to their full capacity.

Negative effects of hunched posture

A hunched posture can make you ill because it means that any physical activity is carried out from a position that accelerates the effects of wear on all of the joints, particularly the structures of the vertebral column. Daily pressure from repeated, asymmetrical sequences of everyday movements is heightened by individual pressure peaks as, for example, when carrying heavy objects while moving house.

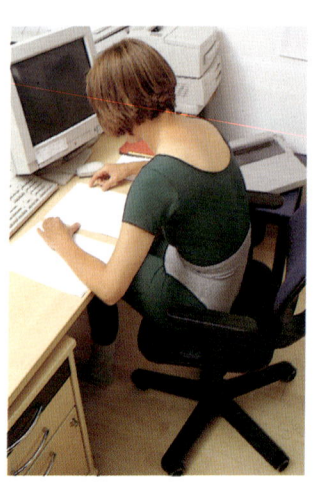

Physical structures are unevenly loaded and therefore more easily damaged

Asymmetrical pressure on the vertebral column in a hunched position means that excessive pressure is applied to the front of the vertebrae and the disks. The other side of the disks, however, is subject to tension. This can lead to tearing on the outside of the ring of fibre so that the gelatinous core of the disk slips out. This is known as a "slipped disk" (see page 32).

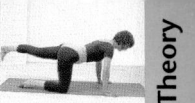

The hunched posture is not only a bad influence on the back, however. Body posture places the joints of the trunk and the limbs in a fundamental relationship to one another. With a hunched posture the rest of the joints are badly positioned because of the vertebral column's change in shape. The articular surfaces are not correctly aligned with each other and therefore have a smaller contact area. This then leads to the articular cartilage being subjected to greater stress at specific points, and therefore wearing out faster. Over the years, this can lead to increased wear and tear (arthritis) of the joints.

Joint surfaces are not correctly aligned

In reverse, because of the mutual interdependence of all parts of the body, a disturbance or defect in the extremities can also have an effect on the back. A foot defect – such as, for example, a splay foot – may in this way have a damaging effect on the position of the knee and therefore even on the hip joint and the vertebral column, because of the changed position of the foot joint. Some people even suffer from headaches caused by a foot defect of this type.

Hunched posture and the resulting altered position of the joints also has a damaging effect on the ligaments stabilizing the joints: some of them are permanently over-extended and others are not subject to any tension at all and cannot therefore fulfil their retaining function. The muscles are similarly under unequal workloads. The back muscles are extended, the stomach and chest muscles, on the other hand, are greatly shortened. In neither of these positions are the muscles able to achieve optimum tension or apply their full strength. This considerably affects the work of the muscles, since this overloading can lead to strain.

Stomach and pectoral muscles are shortened

The most telling example concerns the muscles of the neck and upper back. When the back is hunched, the shoulders slip forward, the arms hang in front of the body and turn in. This means that all the weight of the pectoral girdle and the arms is carried by the muscles of the cervical vertebrae. In addition, the hunched posture

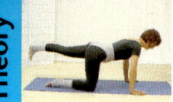

means the head is pushed forward. This is accentuated by sedentary activities that require the head to bend forward, for example reading when sitting down.

Similarly, the load is increased when holding and carrying objects, e.g. when shopping. The neck and

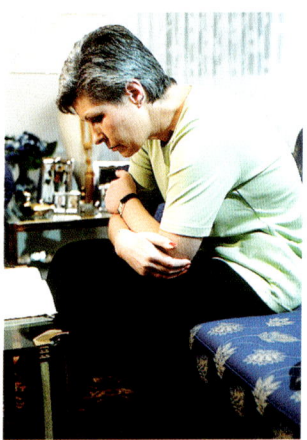

When hunched, the neck and upper back muscles are overloaded

upper back muscles were not designed to carry such heavy weights. The result is strain and, in exceptional cases, upper back syndrome (see page 28).

Cooperation between the different parts of the body

Since it is relatively easy to move the arms and legs independently of the trunk, these can adopt very varied positions in relation to the vertebral column. Many limb positions are favourable to an upright posture, although others are not.

For instance, turning your arms outward makes it easier to raise the ribcage and therefore to adopt an upright position. On the other hand, if the arms are turned inward, it takes more effort to keep the ribcage raised. Therefore, turning the arms inward tends to lead to a hunched back.

Awareness exercise
Either sitting or standing, hold your arms in front of your body, turned inward, and try to raise your ribcage and push it upward and forward.

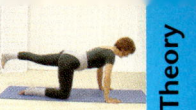

Now repeat the same exercise with your arms on either side of your body, turning outward. Can you feel the enormous difference?

The everyday movements of the arms and hands frequently involve turning them inward: for example, grasping and holding objects, writing by hand or with a typewriter or computer keyboard, and many other manual activities. It is an effort to maintain an upright position while carrying out these arm movements.

To make it easier to adopt an upright position, you should tend to turn your arms outward more. This means, when sitting, that you should place them on either side of you, on the arms of the chair, or squarely on the table. When standing, the arms turn outward more if you put them in your pockets. On the other hand, if the arms are crossed over the upper trunk, they are turning inward; this also means that the shoulders are pulled forward.

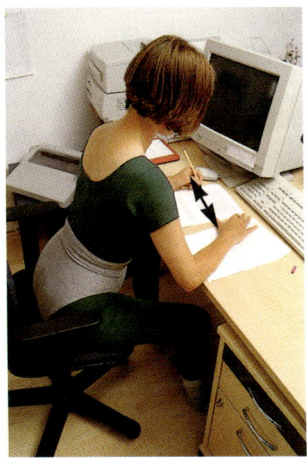

Leaning on widely spread arms promotes an upright posture

Besides the arms, the position of the legs also has a decisive effect on body posture. When sitting, an upright position is encouraged if the legs are apart and the whole of the foot is flat on the floor. This helps to tilt the pelvis forward. Crossed legs, on the other hand, make it almost impossible to straighten the body, or at least make it much more difficult. Women's clothing in particular – among other things, short tight skirts – makes placing the legs slightly apart something of a problem, therefore making it difficult to attain an upright posture.

It seems that many everyday movements encourage posture with poor load distribution. But, if these are not habitual, they need not have a damaging effect. The risk of illness nevertheless increases if movements are frequently carried out with poor posture and hence overloading.

Three golden rules for your back
- Reduce the periods of time when your back is hunched. To start with, pick out specific situations where your posture could be improved.
- Change your everyday environment so that an upright posture becomes easier. Practise common sequences of movements with an upright posture to make them automatic.
- Improve your posture – particularly in demanding circumstances, even if these happen only rarely. This can limit the damaging effects of dangerous overloads.

Common causes of back pain

Back pain may have various causes

The central role of the back for body posture and movement means that back pain may originate in very different parts of the body. It can come from a wide range of muscles and tendons, the joints or even the internal organs. As a result of these different causes, it can also take many different forms.

Back pain may either be restricted to one spot, radiate out to other areas or "move" from one place to another. Stabbing or pulling pain has a different effect from dull or pressing pain.

Typical symptoms are easy to identify. The *exact* cause of the pain should, however, only be diagnosed after a thorough medical examination. Because of the confusing variety of possible causes for back pain, we list in the pages that follow only the problems and diseases

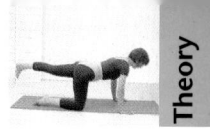

that occur relatively frequently, and where individual action by the patient can have a positive effect on the problem and its symptoms.

Important
If you have back pain or problems with your back that do not disappear on their own, or if the pains keep coming back, it is *essential* that you consult a doctor before trying to treat yourself. The doctor will be able to diagnose the cause and prescribe the correct treatment.

Bad posture

Only in very few cases does defective posture have anything to do with a disease of the vertebral column – it is generally muscular in origin. Muscles that are too weak or that are used asymmetrically lead to poor posture which is intensified by habit and the everyday environment. The muscles adapt over the course of time, some of them shortening and others becoming inactive. This is how hump backs (cyphose) and, more rarely, hollow backs (hyperlodosis) are caused. If, in addition to this, asymmetrical activity is engaged in, or the posture twists frequently to one side, a transverse curvature of the vertebral column (scoliose) may also occur. Carrying a school bag on one side, for example, may intensify this problem.

Posture defects are generally muscular in origin

Hump back: cyphose
In a humped back the vertebral column has changed shape from the normal double curves of the S-shape in the pectoral and lumbar vertebrae to the single curve of the humped back. The ribcage has sunken inward, the shoulders hang forward. The arms turn inward and tend to hang in front of the body; the head is pushed forward.

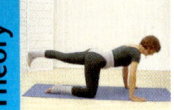

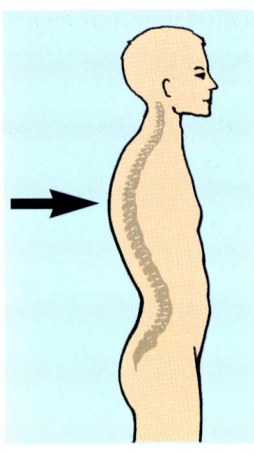

A hump back: the hunched back becomes permanent

This posture is seen frequently, since the force of gravity pulls the body into this position. In addition, almost all day-to-day activity is carried out in front of us and many hand movements encourage a hunched posture (see page 18). During everyday activities, the muscles that pull the body into a hunched position are overloaded and shortened. The muscles that pull us upright find it difficult, or even impossible, to work against this pull forward. This is how a hunched posture becomes established.

Some serious illnesses may also be also associated with a hump back. These include Scheuermann's disease (a developmental problem of the vertebral column during childhood), Bechterew's disease (a chronic inflammation of the joints involving the immune system) and osteoporosis (see page 34).

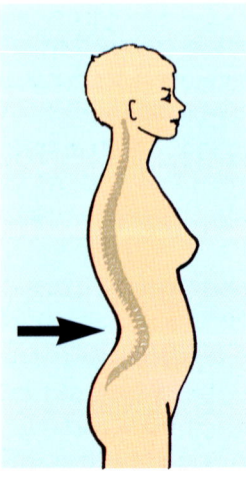

A hollow back can be caused by pregnancy

Hollow back: hyperlodosis

Hollow back is a postural defect at the level of the lumbar vertebrae. The normal inward arch of the lower curve in the vertebral column is exaggerated and the pelvic tilt forward is unnaturally pronounced. However, genuine occurrences of hollow back are much rarer than is generally supposed. The symptoms are often accompanied by excessive rounding of the pectoral vertebrae and are

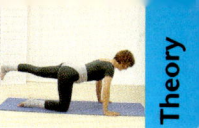

therefore very obvious. When the pectoral vertebrae are straightened, the lumbar vertebrae often lose their hunched shape automatically.

A hollow back may also appear during pregnancy as the greater weight of the stomach pulls the lumbar vertebrae forward. In addition, wearing high heels pushes the pelvis forward unnaturally, causing the development of a hollow back.

Curvature of the spine: scoliosis
The term scoliosis describes a sideways curve in the vertebral column, where the individual vertebrae also twist away from each other. The cause of this is generally not known. Medical causes such as developmental problems, polio or the asymmetrical pull from a scar are fairly rare. More frequent causes are asymmetry in the area of the legs (different leg lengths) or the pelvis.

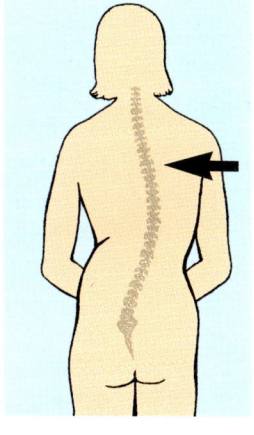

Scoliosis mainly appears during growth

Some scoliotic problems with posture may originate in the womb, if the embryo always lies on one side. In infancy, this preference for one side may be reflected in the often different rates of development of the two sides of the brain. Habitual one-sided posture and movement in children and adults in everyday life is a source of further unequal muscle development, thus exaggerating the sideways curve.
With "true" scoliosis, the asymmetrical, twisted vertebrae are visible in X-rays. In young people there is a particular danger of the defect being exaggerated during growth. Once the bones have stopped growing, the process comes to a halt.

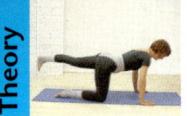

What treatment is there for defective posture?

With all posture defects, an upright posture and therefore the extension of the vertebral column should be encouraged. Symmetrical posture and movement is particularly important with scoliosis.

If there is an anatomical problem of different leg lengths, this must be compensated for with raised shoe heels or soles. In many cases a specially designed corset or surgery are used to prevent further deterioration of the scoliosis if it is already well developed.

Note

If you suspect that your back pain is caused by one of the defective postures described here, go and see your doctor. He or she will give you a precise diagnosis. This is especially important if the back pain involves children and young people who have not yet finished growing.

What to do about defective posture:

- posture training (see page 39)
- changing your everyday and working environments (see page 53)
- relief treatments (see page 84)
- endurance training in sports that are kind to the back and promote physical symmetry (see page 76)
- remedial exercises.

Strengthening the stomach muscles – a common misunderstanding

In the past, strengthening the stomach muscles was often prescribed as a treatment for defective posture, particularly hollow back. This is explained by the fact that the stomach becomes slack and curves outward

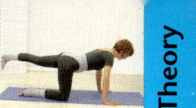

with a hunched posture and so it also appears weak. While strengthening the stomach muscles does eliminate hollow back, the simple act of toning and strengthening the stomach muscles also has the effect of pulling the pelvis and ribcage together. The ribcage sinks inward, the shoulders pull forward and the hunching of the pectoral vertebrae increases. In this way, the hunched posture is not compensated for but encouraged.

Shortened stomach muscles pull the pelvis and the ribcage together

To support the upright posture, on the other hand, the pelvis and the ribcage must be separated. To do this, the stomach muscles have to be lengthened. This will make the stomach flatter and the waist narrower. Lifting the ribcage flattens the hollow back, so that the vertebral column adopts its normal S-curves. The function of the stomach muscles is to stabilize, but they need to be long: this effect can be achieved through stretching exercises.

While strengthening exercises appear to be right for the stomach muscles, the stress must be on stabilization through long muscles. It is essential to correct the vertebral column, straighten it during the exercises and make sure that the long stomach muscles separate the pelvis and ribcage (see page 68). The load on the vertebral column is at its lowest in this position. The usual stomach exercises – "crunches" or "sit-ups" – bring the pelvis and ribcage together, the vertebral column becomes rounded and the stomach muscles shorten.

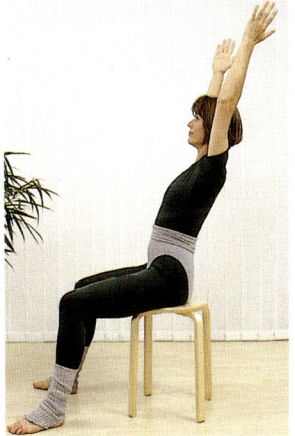

Purpose of strengthening the stomach muscles: targeting a stable upright posture

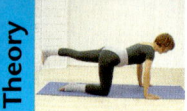

Back strain/stiffness

Back strain is the most frequent of all back problems. Pulling pains in the neck and upper back and between the shoulder blades, a feeling of pressure on the breastbone and radiating pains in one or both arms are typical. This is known as the upper back (UB) syndrome (see page 28).

If you have pain after standing or sitting for a long time, or when bending over, it is likely that you have a problem with the lower vertebrae, or the so-called lower back (LB) syndrome.

The causes of strain may be your everyday posture or the leisure activities in which you take part. This is especially true if your movement is one-sided and overloads specific areas of the body and muscles. People

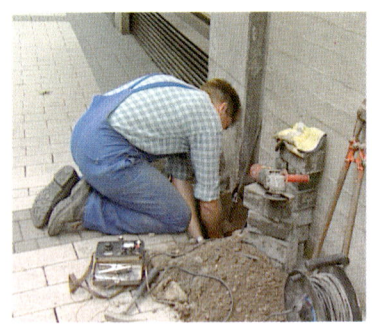

Poor posture at work often causes strain

who engage in physical work every day – for example, lifting and carrying heavy weights on site or in a workshop – or who work in draughty or damp places or use their arms asymmetrically on a conveyor belt, suffer from back and shoulder pain as part of their "normal" everyday life. But conditions are just as damaging for people who spend the whole day sitting or standing – for example at the till in a supermarket, in front of a computer or at a drawing board.

Even after work, the body is not always allowed to rest. Sports such as tennis and badminton, which place asymmetrical demands on the body, may exaggerate the unequal demands that already exist at work. Strenuous sports such as rowing and team games may place excessive strain on the muscles, particularly if they are already under stress or have not had the right training.

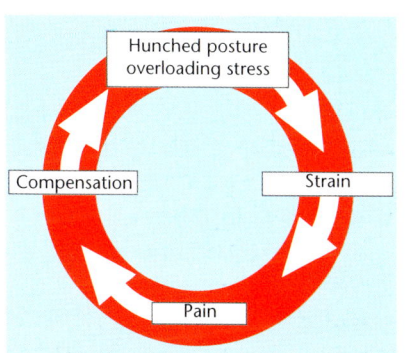

Even power training can cause strain if you demand too much of yourself during specific exercises and do them incorrectly and/or without proper guidance from a qualified trainer. Back strain may also quickly occur as the result of unaccustomed, asymmetrical actions in the house and garden, or when doing DIY.

One factor that considerably increases the risk of back strain is a hunched posture. This bent-over posture with a rounded back and changed position of the joints causes additional uneven loading on the muscles. The body registers this and attempts to take corrective action by activating the relevant muscles. However, the muscles are unable to draw on their full capacity when the body is in a hunched position (see page 17). The compensatory muscle action, therefore, requires a constant output of unnaturally high levels of energy. If the type of everyday activity described above is added to this, there will be problems in store.

The body defends itself against a hunched back

Another frequent cause of back strain, and problems associated with physical over-exertion, is mental stress. In addition to professional and personal worries, the causes may well also lie in general personality problems (see page 36).

If the causes of strain are not recognized and treated, a vicious circle is formed with hunched posture, over-exertion, and stress leading to back strain. This causes pain. The pain heightens the mental stress and leads to "compensatory behaviour." This in its turn heightens the muscle pain and causes more back strain.

Hunched posture overloading stress

Compensation

Strain

Pain

Vicious circle of strain

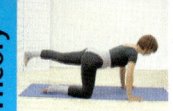

What treatment is there?

Looking at the causes of back strain described here, it is apparent that there is every possibility that those who are affected can take some control over the pain. First, it is important to trace the cause of the strain. Successful treatment depends entirely on awareness of the role played by a hunched posture, physical overload, asymmetrical activities and mental stress. Remedial measures can only be taken once the causes have been properly recognized.

The following measures are recommended, depending on the cause:

- posture training (see page 39)
- changing the everyday and working environments (see page 53)
- endurance training in sports that are kind to the back (see page 76)
- relief postures (see page 81)
- relief remedies (see page 84)
- home heat-treatment remedies (see page 85)
- relaxation (see page 80)
- psychological counselling or psychotherapy (see page 37).

Upper back syndrome

If your cervical vertebrae crack when you move, migraine-type headaches begin and the neck and upper back muscles are strained, if you have pain radiating through your shoulder and arm or restricted head movement, you have upper back (UB) syndrome. The cause of these problems is almost always a hunched posture. The pectoral girdle slips forward on to the ribcage and the whole weight of the pectoral girdle and the arms is borne by the neck and upper back muscles. These were not designed for this type of work and are overloaded. Stress factors caused by the increased muscle

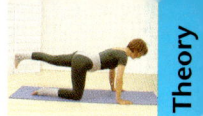

tension may make the situation considerably worse. In many cases impairment of the foot and hand muscles may also lead to UB syndrome. Twisting or over-exertion of finger or hand muscles (for instance when knitting) may also be responsible. The neck and upper back muscles are then activated in reaction to this: i.e. the pain appears at a point other than where the problem lies. If you think this is the case, try the stretching exercises no.

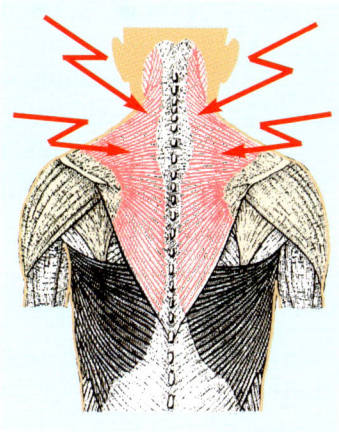

Radiating pain and restricted movement are indicators of upper back syndrome

1 (see page 57) and no. 10 (see page 63) described in the practical section of this book.

What treatment is there?

The painful side-effects of upper back syndrome can be ameliorated in the short term with various home remedies (see page 85). For a permanent solution to the problem of back strain, the cause of the muscle overload must be removed; this means that, in most cases, training must be given for upright posture and the everyday environment must be changed to encourage the elimination of poor posture.

Measures for treating upper back syndrome:
- posture training (see page 39)
- changing the everyday and working environments (see page 53)
- endurance training in sports that are kind to the back and promote physical symmetry (see page 76)
- relief postures (see page 81)
- relief remedies (see page 84)
- relaxation (see page 80)
- physiotherapy treatment.

Lumbago

The pain caused by lumbago is not easily forgotten. It shoots through "bone and marrow" completely unexpectedly when you are bending or lifting something. It's almost unbearable to move at all and no relief can be gained by either sitting or lying down.

Also known as acute back strain, the pain is comparable to the after-effects of a slipped disk. The difference is that, on close examination, no physical symptoms can be detected.

This means that lumbago is one of the "functional" diseases that cause no physical changes in the body. Over-exertion of the muscles is responsible for lumbago. The stomach muscles are often affected, for example when they have to work in unfavourable conditions when the back is hunched. Irritation occurs at the connection between the muscle and bone in the area of the pubic bone. The pain caused in the affected muscle does not, however, appear at the point of origin but is often felt in the back. Relief is often achieved by lying on the back with the knees bent, as the stomach muscles are then in a resting position. A warm hot-water bottle on the lower stomach can help to relieve the pain.

Overworked muscles cause lumbago

What treatment is there?

Measures to relieve the pain:
- relief postures (see page 81)
- relief remedies (see page 84)
- home heat-treatment remedies (see page 85)
- physiotherapy treatments.

Preventative measures:
- posture training (see page 39)
- changing the everyday and the working environments (see page 53)
- endurance training in sports that are kind to the back and promote physical symmetry (see page 76).

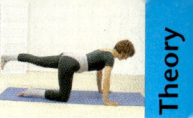

Damaged vertebrae

Age-related problems are just as common in the vertebrae and disks as in any other of the body's structures as one gets older. The rate of the aging process is nevertheless strongly influenced by the nature and frequency of the demands placed upon the body. A lifelong hunched back will lead to rapid erosion of the vertebrae and disks. An upright posture, on the other hand, will not damage these structures.

Accelerated damage with a hunched posture

It is mainly the small vertebral joints and the disks that are affected by signs of deterioration. The most obvious signs are in the two more mobile sections of the vertebral column: the cervical and lumbar sections. The earliest signs of damage are usually strain and stiffness when moving.

What treatment is there?

As in so many instances, but specifically regarding damage, prevention is better than cure. It is the everyday stress that causes the aging process to accelerate and the type and intensity of this stress that influences the timescale and speed of wear.

Measures to prevent vertebral erosion and to slow down the aging process:
- posture training (see page 39)
- changing the everyday and the working environments (see page 53)
- endurance training in sports that are kind to the back and promote physical symmetry (see page 76)
- relief remedies (see page 84).

Damaged joints

Like the vertebral column, the body's joints are also susceptible to the aging process. Physical work, asymmetrical working positions with a hunched back, and being overweight, can accelerate the normal aging process. This affects the knee and hip joints particularly frequently. Wear and tear can lead to painful inflammation of the joints. The "initial pain" is typical of this type of "arthritic joint:" movement becomes easier only after it has been repeated several times and the stiffness and pain disappear only slowly. People change their posture to take the strain off the damaged, painful joint. To do this, muscles throughout the body are mobilized and the resulting physiological imbalance may lead to back pain.

Arthritic pain leads to compensatory posture

What treatment is there?

A healthy everyday life, the right physical compensation and an upright posture help to distribute the optimum load to correctly positioned joints, to maintain condition and therefore prevent signs of deterioration. If arthritis is present, various home remedies (such as heat-packs applied to the affected areas) can help to relieve the pain (see page 85).

Measures to prevent damage to the joints:
- posture training (see page 39)
- changing the everyday and working environments (see page 53)
- sports that are kind to the back (see page 76)
- relief remedies (see page 84).

Slipped disk

As the name suggests, with a slipped disk the gelatinous core of the disk "slips," i.e. it pushes out between the

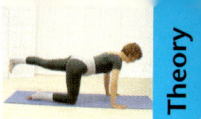

two vertebrae. This may happen if the disk's outer fibrous ring becomes inflexible and tears, so that the inside contents can push through (see page 9).

In most cases it is the disks in the lumbar region that are affected as this is where the most powerful forces are at work. The section of the disk that has slipped out generally presses on one of the

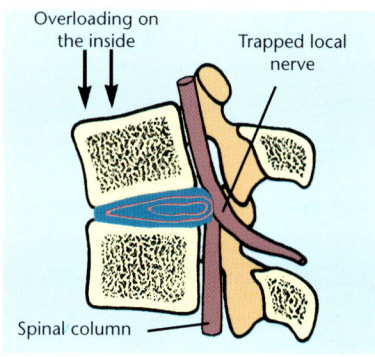

The core of a disk that has slipped and is pressing on a nerve

nerves that branches out from the spinal column between the vertebrae. The nerves that are affected in the lumbar region connect the spinal column with the legs, so that a slipped disk here causes pain and can even be crippling. In rarer cases, the disks in the cervical vertebrae are affected and the problems then occur in one of the arms. A slipped disk is triggered in the same way as an attack of lumbago, generally by a sideways or twisting, bending, or lifting movement. The pain, known as sciatica, is similar to lumbago. It occurs suddenly and can shoot down as far as the legs. Afterwards, very little movement is possible and only specific compensating positions can bring any relief. If nerves are affected, the leg generally has no strength. The results may be lameness and numbness of the skin. In some cases symptoms may also include problems with the bowel and the bladder, and the affected individual has no control over defecation and urination.

In the worst cases the result is lameness

What treatment is there?
If lumbago-like pain occurs, always see your doctor just to rule out the possibility of a slipped disk. If you get to the stage where you go lame, feel numb and have bowel

and bladder problems, a visit to the doctor is essential as there is a risk of permanent nerve damage.

The following treatments may be tried, provided a doctor has first been consulted. At this point we must emphasize that you should only continue with any of these posture training and strengthening exercises as long as you feel no pain; stop doing them immediately if the pain returns or worsens.

Measures to alleviate pain with a slipped disk:
- relaxation (see page 80)
- relief postures (see page 81)
- relief remedies (see page 84)
- home heat-treatment remedies (see page 85)
- physiotherapy treatment.

Preventative measures:
- posture training (see page 39)
- changing the everyday and working environments (see page 53).

Osteoporosis

Decisive: bone development during growth

Bone quality deteriorates with increasing age. It becomes more porous and is less stable as the aging process sets in. But this process accelerates at different speeds with every individual. If bone development is given optimum support through nutritious food and a lot of activity while a young person is growing, the point when age-related bone deterioration becomes a problem is delayed and the risk of suffering from osteoporosis is reduced. Conditions are favourable for osteoporosis when there is little activity and this is exacerbated by hormonal irregularities. Even in youth, this type of irregularity may have a negative effect on bone development. The worst damage affects young sports competitors and young people who suffer from anorexia and are seriously underweight. The hormonal changes after a woman's menopause (change of life) have a similar effect,

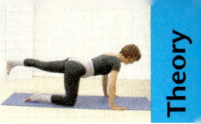
accelerating the rate of bone deterioration. That's why women are more frequently affected by this condition than are men. Finally, excessive alcohol, caffeine and nicotine consumption also creates favourable conditions for osteoporosis.

Hormones influence bone metabolism

The changes in the bones occur gradually and are not felt at first. Even in X-rays, the condition only becomes apparent when there is already an increased danger of broken bones. The first obvious problems are usually back pains that may also "travel" to other parts of the body. When the customary posture is a hunched back, which places unequal pressure on the vertebral column, the vertebrae may, in the advanced stage, even break into wedge-shaped pieces without any extra pressure being exerted. A permanent hump back is formed in this way. All the other bones are at risk of breaking as well – the upper thighbones, for example. The pain is mainly caused by the severe strain that occurs if some muscles are overloaded through a change in posture.

Pain through strain

What treatment is there?

To prevent bones from breaking, an upright posture should always be maintained in order to protect the vertebral column.

> Exercises to encourage an upright posture must only be followed with caution if you have osteoporosis and should only be continued if there is no pain. *Stop immediately if you feel any pain.*

Moderate but regular sport which is kind to the back will harden the bones, improve mobility and dexterity as well as muscle endurance. These are measures that prevent bone deterioration and can therefore be recommended for people of any age. With older patients the intensity of the movements must be appropriate to their physical condition. If the problem already exists, the everyday environment should be adapted to take into account the increased risk of breaking bones.

Measures to prevent osteoporosis and breakages:
- posture training (see page 39)
- changing the everyday and working environments (see page 53)
- sports that are kind to the back (see page 76)
- correct diet.

Additional measures for pain relief and slowing the spread of the condition:
- relief postures (see page 81)
- relief remedies (see page 84)
- home heat-treatment remedies (see page 85)
- physiotherapy treatment
- medication prescribed by a doctor.

Diseases of the internal organs

Internal disease may cause back pain

Back pain may also lead to diseases of the internal organs. Among these, for example, are inflammation of the lungs, heart disease, bowel problems, and kidney disease. The treatments for these are very different, depending on the condition, and are directed less at the back than at the organs concerned. We will not, therefore, describe them here.

However, if you have chronic pain that is difficult to control, it would be sensible to have your internal organs examined by your physician.

Psychosomatic back pain

A frequent cause of back pain, which is often underestimated by orthopaedic practitioners, is "mental stress." Even without any additional physical stress it is possible for psychological problems and changes in hormone levels to cause psychosomatic conditions in

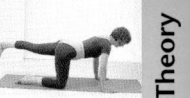

the back. These generally begin as painful back strain from which upper back or lower back syndrome may later develop.

The fact that our physical and mental well-being are closely connected, and often interdependent, is even reflected in the way we speak. People who are constantly under pressure, who always appear "to have a set mouth," "to be tearing their hair out" and even "to be as stiff as a board," suffer more frequently from physical strain than those people who are able to allow their emotions a little more expression.

The physical and mental condition of the individual are interconnected

It is mainly the chronic tensions lying under the surface that can be a cause of continuing back problems. Transient problems that are affected by the environment, such as unemployment and excessive hours of work, are just as much to blame as problems with a partner or within the family.

Not least are the effects of personality problems such as an inferiority complex, a lack of self-confidence or fear: these may all be expressed in the form of back pain. In such cases, back pain may also be unconsciously "used" by the sufferer as a means of avoiding the more intense emotional pain of examining the cause or the effort of changing the environment.

What treatment is there?

Psychological treatments must be central in looking for the causes of psychosomatic back problems. Relaxation training, combined with training in posture and physical compensation, is best suited to combating stress but is not adequate for handling serious personality problems. Various forms of psycho-therapy are, however, available, depending on the complexity of the problems. The prerequisite for this is that the individuals concerned take the initia-tive themselves and decide they really want to sort out these sometimes difficult problems. In the United States as in Western Europe, consultations with a therapist and long-term psychoanalysis are a recognized

Psychology is a central consideration

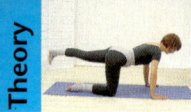
part of the health insurance process if an illness has been diagnosed. In this respect, back problems may also be considered an illness.

Measures against psychosomatic back problems:
- psychological counselling or psychotherapy
- relaxation (see page 80).

Supportive measures:
- posture training (see page 39)
- changing the everyday and working environments (see page 53)
- sports that are kind to the back (see page 76).

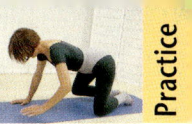

II. Practice: How to keep your back fit

The following section contains detailed descriptions of how you can strengthen your back and keep it strong enough for an upright posture. You will learn how to adopt the right posture during your everyday activities, how to make your muscles work with stretching and strengthening exercises, which sports are kind to the back and strengthen it and which home remedies you can use for relaxation and relief.

How to use the book and video together when exercising

If you have already studied the basics in the "Theory" section and watched the video, you will already have a very good picture of the exercises described in this practical section. While reading through, you can watch any exercises you find difficult on the video again. The camera icon next to the individual exercises will help you to find the right video sequence by using the minute-counter on your video recorder. Simply set the counter to zero (display in minutes) when you insert the tape and fast-forward it to the figure given beside the camera icon.

Posture training

 1:35

Getting up and lying down

1:50

To stand up, many people roll their upper body upward from the prone position. This puts a great deal of pressure on the vertebrae and disks.

A more reasonable starting point if you want to be kind to your back when getting up, is to turn on to your side first. That is, while still lying down, turn on to your

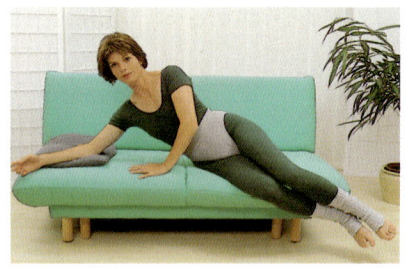

**Getting up:
always from
the side**

side, bend your knees slightly and, stretching your arms upward, raise yourself sideways into a sitting position. You can move your legs from the bed to the floor at the same time. This way, the upper body remains straight. To lie down, do the same movements in reverse.

2:05 🎥

Sitting down

The position of the legs

Use a chair with a flat seat. The height of the seat should

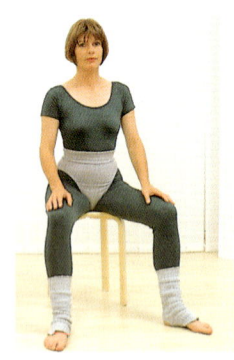

**Placing the
legs widely
apart**

be at least as high as your lower leg, so that your thighs are parallel to the floor or slope slightly down to the knee. Sit on the front half of the seat, with your feet flat on the floor. Set your legs slightly apart, so that you can stand up without losing your balance. Place your ankle joints vertically below the knees. Looking down at one leg, you can now follow the line of the leg. It traverses the thigh, goes over the knee to the ankle joint and continues to the big toe. The leg should form a continual straight line: this is to ensure that working conditions for the knee and ankle joints are correct and that the leg and foot muscles can contribute to maintaining an upright posture.

The pelvic tilt

When the back is hunched, the pelvis and the lumbar vertebrae roll back. However, it is necessary to tilt the pelvis forward and downward for an upright posture. Put

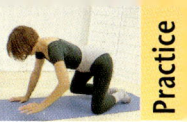
your hands on your hips and move your pelvis forward and back – you will feel clearly how the pelvis moves. If you sit on a hard seat you will feel the two ischia bones when you do this. Now find out at which

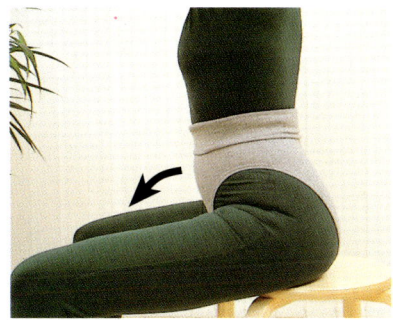

Pelvis tilting forward and downward

point of this movement you feel these two bones most strongly against the seat. Tilt the pelvis just a little further forward. This makes the ischia move back, but you will still be able to feel them slightly. Take note of this position for your pelvis. The lumbar vertebrae are now correctly aligned.

Raising the ribcage

Place one hand on your lower stomach and the other on your breastbone. With a hunched back your hands will be close together. If you now tilt your pelvis forward and downward, your hands will separate a little. Now raise your ribcage upward and outward. At the same time, imagine that a thread is attached to your breastbone and is pulling you

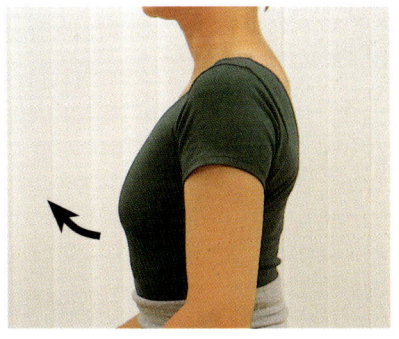

Ribcage raised upward and outward

upward and outward. Do not pull your shoulders up as well, but allow them to rest loosely on either side. It is also important not to press your shoulder blades together or to lean back. If you allow your arms to hang down by your body, the pectoral girdle, viewed from the side, will now be somewhere in

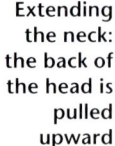
the middle, over the ribcage. Now rest your hands on top of your thighs.

Extending the neck

Imagine that a thread attached to the back of the head is pulling you up even more. This will extend the neck

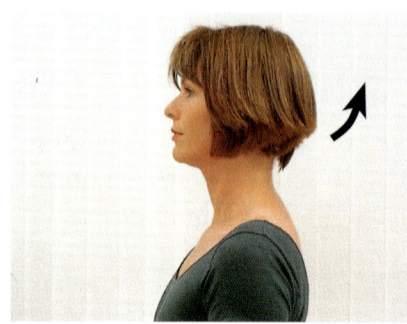

so that it becomes longer. Your head is now in a straight line with the vertebral column and your chin is closer to the neck. You are now sitting with an upright posture.

Extending the neck: the back of the head is pulled upward

Upright posture while sitting:
- tilt your pelvis forward and downward
- raise your ribcage upward and outward
- extend your neck
- place your feet slightly apart and flat on the floor
- your shoulders rest loosely at either side.

When you are practising the upright sitting position, concentrate initially on one section of the body at a time, correct this, then go on to the next. After a few tries you should be able to tilt your pelvis, raise your ribcage and extend your neck simultaneously, because the correct alignment of the vertebral column is the natural outcome of all this. Of course, in the upright sitting position you may also turn your head freely in any direction.

An upright posture is difficult to start with

If you usually sit in a hunched position, you will probably feel that the upright posture is difficult and requires concentration. This is quite natural, as the muscles adapt themselves to a customary hunched posture. Many of them are shortened and others are

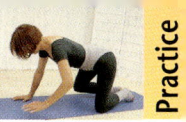

hardly used (see page 17). You can imagine that, as soon as you are upright, you will be pulled back into the hunched posture by the shortened muscles as if they were rubber bands. You will therefore have to give these muscles some time to get used to this new situation: some of the muscles must get longer and others that were hardly active at all before must suddenly start working again.

Shortened muscles work like rubber bands

To achieve an upright posture successfully, it is essential that you can feel in your own body how much straighter you really could be. The posture should be demanding, but should not cause pain or cramps.

You should also remember that your body was not designed to remain in the same position for long periods of time. So please don't force yourself to sit for hours in the upright position. If it isn't possible to change positions, you could at least relieve your muscles of some of the work by using some of the relief measures described on page 84.

Everyday awareness exercise

Take time out every day to take stock of your sitting position. What position is your pelvis in, your ribcage, your pectoral girdle and your head? Try to straighten your posture. Hold this position for a while, without feeling any twinges. Only use as much muscle power as is really needed.

Regular awareness exercises will help you on the way to achieving to an upright posture. They apply the right pressure to the muscles and the length of time you spend sitting in a hunched position every day will get shorter without your having to spend extra time on the problem.

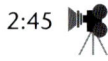

2:45

Standing and walking

After you have learned how to maintain an upright posture sitting down, it is not difficult to do the same thing standing up.

Place your feet hip-width apart. Point the toes slightly outward, a bit like clock hands pointing at ten to two. Flex the knee joints a little, making sure they are not locked straight. As when sitting, tilt the pelvis forward and downward and the ribcage upward and outward. To feel this movement properly, place one hand on your lower stomach and the other hand on the breastbone.

Tilt the pelvis and raise the ribcage, as when sitting

In a hunched position, as we have seen, the distance between the two hands is shorter than in the upright posture. Take particular care when raising the ribcage. If the pelvis is tilted on its own, but the ribcage is still sunk in, the lumbar vertebrae will shift to form a hollow back (see page 22).

On the other hand, if the pelvis and ribcage move at the same time, the vertebral column is extended and correctly realigned. Remember: to raise the ribcage, lift the breastbone and don't pull the shoulders back.

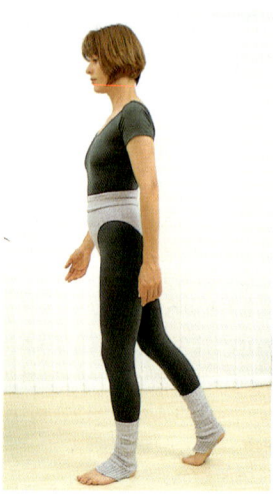

Turn the feet slightly outward, let the arms swing loosely

Now begin to walk, swinging your arms loosely by your sides. The main features of the upright posture when walking are the slightly outward turn of the feet and the raised ribcage. A slow amble will encourage a hunched posture. On the other hand, a fast walk makes the upright posture easier. This is why a good walking speed is somewhere in the range of 80–120 paces a minute. The advantage of the

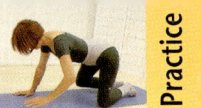

upright posture is that, when you are walking, less energy is expended than with a hunched back. With the latter, the legs drag the body along behind them. When you are upright, on the other hand, the breastbone takes the lead so that you walk almost automatically.

Lead with the breastbone

Just like sitting upright, walking upright cuts down the time you spend every day in a hunched position. It helps the vertebral column to stay healthy and keeps it in good condition.

Upright posture for standing and walking:
- tilt your pelvis forward and downward
- raise your ribcage upward and outward
- extend your neck
- turn your feet slightly outward
- swing your arms loosely by your sides.

Bending, lifting, and carrying

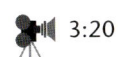 3:20

Bending and lifting movements put some of the heaviest pressure on the vertebral column. However, they are found repeatedly in everyday actions – getting up and sitting down, vacuuming, washing your hair at the edge of the bath, and working in the kitchen, to name just a few examples. Depending on the frequency and intensity of the workload, bending and lifting causes most cases of lumbago and slipped disks (see pages 30 and 32).

Bending

Have a look at weight-lifters to see how they perform bending and lifting movements, placing minimum strain on the back. The legs are placed more than shoulder-width apart and are turned slightly outward. The pelvis tilts forward and the ribcage is raised. From this position, the process begins by bending at both the hips and the knees simultaneously. At the same time,

Imagine a weight-lifter

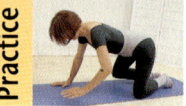

the upper body bends forward, but remains straight. It stops in an oblique position, or almost horizontal, depending on how low you want to bend.

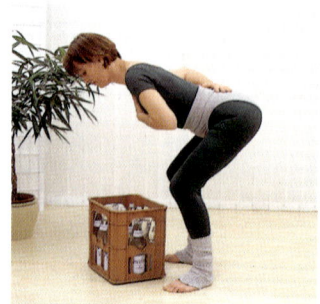

Bend at the knees and hips, keeping the back straight

To practise this movement, adopt the upright standing posture. Place one hand on the breastbone and the other on the lower back, at the level of the lumbar vertebrae. You can now feel whether the pelvis is still tilting forward and the breastbone is raised. Now bend over a few times, bending at the knees and the hips but keeping the back straight. Ideally, you should watch yourself in a mirror. Slowly try to see how far you can bend over without your back hunching. Note where this happens and look for something the same height in your home. The correct movement is easier to practise using this object as a guide.

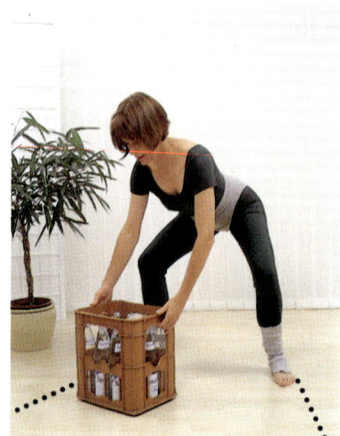

The "work area" is between lines extending from each leg

Bending to the side is even more damaging than bending forward wrongly, because it twists the vertebral column in addition to bending it. To prevent this, you should keep to a "work area" when bending and lifting, and restrict this to the area in front of you. Your legs form the outside limits and, inside this work area, the vertebral column is in optimum alignment for bending movements. Movements

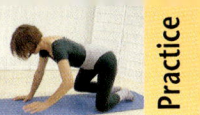
that extend to the sides, beyond the limits of the leg lines, will involve excessive workloads. You can feel this if you try these movements out. The more you turn to the side when bending, the more energy the back must expend to maintain the position of the upper body. This involves intensive one-sided pressure being applied to the disks of the lower spine. Instead of a sideways twist, the work area should preferably be shifted by taking a few steps to one side, as required.

The greater the turn, the heavier the loading

Upright posture when bending:

- tilt your pelvis forward and downward
- raise your ribcage upward and outward
- extend your neck
- place your legs more than shoulder-width apart and bend at the hips and knees
- your back is straight
- the "work area" is defined by a line extending forward from each leg.

If you have to bend very low – for instance, if you are lifting something from the floor – strength is improved by placing one foot slightly back or one knee on the floor. This will make the upright posture easier for the back. For floor-level activity such as weeding, you may also kneel down; a cushion under the knees will help to protect them.

Place one leg behind the other

Lifting

The load on the vertebral column caused by bending is increased when something heavy is being picked up at the same time. You should therefore take special care to maintain good posture when lifting and carrying.

To lift an object, you generally need to bend first. When doing this, remember that the hips and the knees should bend, as just described, but not the back. Before lifting an object, pull it toward you so that it is positioned between your legs, which are shoulder-width apart. You are now in the initial position for lifting: bending

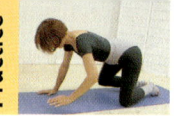
Initial position for lifting

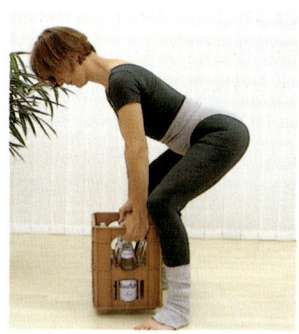

at the knees and hips, upper body straight, eyes looking forward and your outstretched arms and hands holding the object. At the moment of lifting, the ribcage must be raised and the stomach must stay long. This means you will keep your back straight as it takes the load. Lift the object close to the body, with straight arms. At the same time, straighten the hips and knees, slowly at first, and without straightening them completely. Now, if necessary, bend your arms and hold the object in front of your stomach. In this way you will distribute the weight evenly between leg, arm and back muscles.

Straighten knee and hip joints at the same time

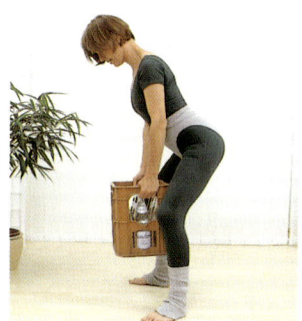

Upright posture while lifting:

- tilt your pelvis forward and downward
- raise your ribcage upward and outward
- extend your neck
- place your legs more than shoulder-width apart and bend at the hips and knees
- keep your back straight
- the "work area" is defined by a line extending forward from each leg
- lift the object close to the body and straighten the hip and knee joints at the same time (but do not straighten completely), keeping your arms bent.

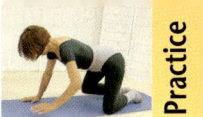

If you do not keep your back straight while lifting, your shoulders will be pulled forward by the weight you are lifting. Your ribcage will then sink and the whole weight will be supported only by the cervical vertebrae. At the same time, the pressure on the disks will increase because of the undesirable curve of the whole vertebral column.

Carrying

Once you have lifted an object in the upright position, it is just as important to have a spine-friendly way of carrying things.

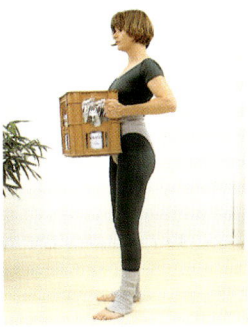

Carry heavy objects close to the body

Carrying things in front of you makes an upright posture difficult because they tend to pull the shoulders forward. If you carry objects in front of you, keep them as close to the body as possible and lift the ribcage.

If you carry objects by your side, it would be better to distribute the weight on both sides so that the pressure on the vertebral column is not one-s.ded. During the years of growth, carrying a heavy school bag may worsen an existing curvature of the spine (scoliosis) (see page 23). Naturally, the load on the vertebral column is all the greater, the heavier the object you are carrying. So avoid weights that are too much for you. If possible, distribute the weight over two trips, or use aids such as rucksacks or shopping trolleys.

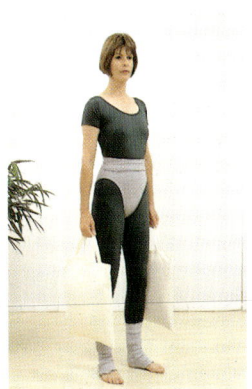

Distribute the weight on both sides

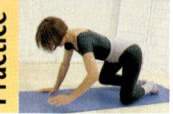

Upright posture when carrying:

- tilt your pelvis forward and downward
- raise your ribcage upward and outward
- extend your neck
- either carry objects close to the body, with arms folded, or
- on both sides of the body.

4:15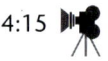

Lying down and sleeping

Muscles recuperate and relax from their daily support work during the long overnight rest period. The pressure on the joints and the disks is reduced and the disks can take up liquid and so regenerate themselves (see page 10).

Each individual prefers their own favorite position when going to sleep. Unfortunately, this is often a position that reflects daytime pressures and habits, i.e. a hunched posture. As movement during sleep is unconscious, it is only possible to specify a position to go to sleep in. If a correct "upright" position is chosen, this will also change over time while we sleep. This is how the holding framework of the body regenerates during the night.

During shorter rest periods, or when you wish to achieve a better result while you rest, you may also opt for a stretching posture (see page 55).

When sleeping, you adopt your customary posture

The positions described in the following sections describe the optimum physical posture when lying down. If these positions are initially uncomfortable, you could change to a more acceptable position later. Even when lying down it is better to be partially straight than not at all.

The best thing for resting and sleeping is a flat bed, with neither a raised head nor foot section. The mattress should neither be too hard nor too soft. The body should be able to sink in a little at the shoulder and pelvic areas

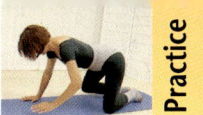
(i.e. at those places that press down most). At the same time, the lumbar and cervical vertebrae should be supported. Latex and foam mattresses have properties like this. A special base is not necessary, but make sure that the mattress is well aired.

The pillows should not be too thick or large. Feather or fibre pillows are suitable as these vary in thickness. If you are lying on your back, they should be thinner, and thicker if you are lying on your side.

Lying on your back

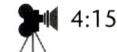 4:15

When lying on your back, it is advisable to use just a thin pillow or cushion. It should be placed under the head only, not under the shoulders. If you prefer, you may support the lower and mid-back with a folded towel. This may still be used if you turn on to your side while sleeping as it will then support the waist.

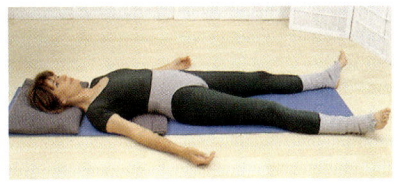

Lying on the back with a thin pillow

Upright posture lying on your back:
- tilt your pelvis forward and downward
- raise your ribcage upward and outward
- extend your neck and support it with a thin pillow.

Lying on your side

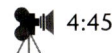 4:45

When lying on your side, bend both your legs slightly at the hips and knees. They can either lie sideways, one on top of the other, or one leg may be stretched out further. Just as when sitting or standing, tilt the pelvis forward, raise the ribcage and extend the neck so that your head

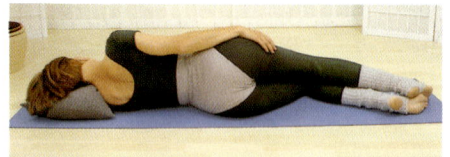

"Upright" side position

prolongs the vertebral column in a straight line and the spine is correctly aligned.

Support your head with a pillow. This should be exactly the height needed for the cervical vertebrae neither to curve sideways and upward nor to sink downward. Push the lower shoulder forward a little and bend the lower arm slightly. The upper arm lies along the side of the body.

Upright posture lying on your side:

- the legs are slightly bent and one on top of the other, or one leg is stretched out
- tilt your pelvis forward and downward
- raise your ribcage upward and outward
- stretch your neck and support it with a pillow
- push the lower shoulder forward a little and bend the lower arm slightly
- the upper arm lies along the side of the body.

5:20 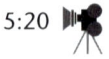 ### Lying on your stomach

Lying on your stomach with your head turned to one side puts an unpleasant strain on your cervical vertebrae. The head is pressed into the bed by the weight of the body, so that the cervical vertebrae are twisted and under pressure. However, with a tiny change in this frontal stomach position, you can improve this awkward posture.

If you wish to lie on your stomach, bend the arm and leg of the side of the body your head is turned toward. This slightly raises that half of the body and the weight is taken off the cervical vertebrae. The arm on the other side should not be pulled in under the stomach but should be to one side, close to the body. For support, you could place a pillow under the upper body on the side the head is facing, from the shoulder to the pelvis. You do not need a pillow for your head in this position.

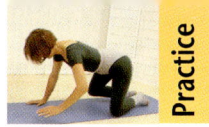

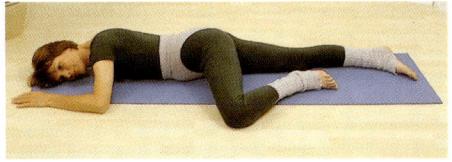

Lying on the stomach with bent arm and leg

Upright posture lying on your stomach:
- tilt your pelvis forward and downward
- raise your ribcage upward and outward
- extend your neck
- bend the arm and leg on the side your head is turned towards; place the other arm by your side, close to the body.

Everyday and work environment

The upright posture becomes easier if your everyday environment matches your physical needs. If, on the other hand, your body has to cope with unsuitable furniture that does not meet your needs, this is another damaging situation. A good look at your environment can reveal that even small changes and remedies can do a lot to maintain a healthy back.

As many people do sedentary work, and the vertebral column is more heavily loaded when sitting than when standing, the correct shape and position of the chair and the work table or desk are particularly important.

The chair should be at least as high as the lower leg. Higher would be better, as the thighs then slope downward slightly to the knee. The seat itself should be flat or slope slightly forward. It must on no account slope back or be hollow in shape. Both of these encourage a hunched position. In addition, the seat must be broad enough to allow the legs to be apart, otherwise an upright posture is seriously restricted.

Make sure your work chair is right

The most suitable backrest follows the shape of the upright vertebral column, i.e. it is slightly curved. This enables it to support and, most importantly, to take the weight at the transition between the lumbar and

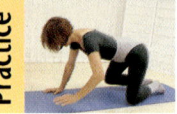
pectoral vertebrae. The optimum height for the backrest depends on the activity involved: if you have to move your arms a lot, the backrest should only come up as far as the shoulder blades. If you are less active, it may even extend as far as the upper back. Upper back support is only useful if you lean back frequently. When doing this, you must not push your head forward into the hunched posture.

Accessories that take the strain off the vertebral column when you are sitting include a cushion for the small of the back (for work with one of these, see page 84) and a wedge cushion (for work with the body leaning forward, see page 85). Occasionally, we recommend "dynamic sitting" on the so-called exercise ball or Pezzi ball. Maintaining an upright posture is quite easy on this type of rubber ball. The increased mobility of the ball simultaneously mobilizes the vertebral column. This is why an exercise ball is a sound investment for any place of work. In your free time, higher seating – such as, for example, bar stools – also helps you to achieve an upright posture.

Lumbar cushion, wedge, exercise ball

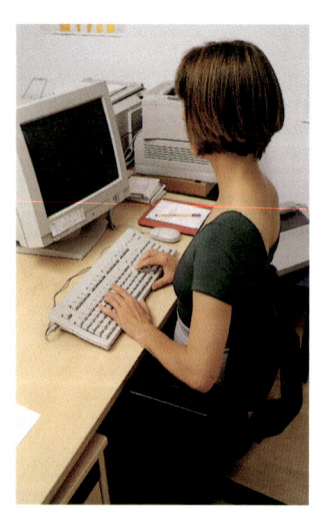

It is important to adapt your working environment to your physical needs

The right height for your work table depends on the height of your seat and the type of activity involved. For reading and writing, with an upright chair and arms slightly spread, the forearms should be able to rest horizontally on the surface. Set the seat slightly higher if you are working on a keyboard.

Select the shape of your desk to suit the work you do. A semi-circular desk provides a wide work area if you can turn your seat. But you must also be able to

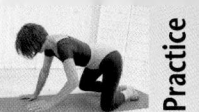

move your legs to either side for this: there must be no drawers in the way.

Once you have carefully analysed your everyday environment and tailored it to your physical requirements, you can now help your body to feel good and to be relaxed in the upright posture. Stretching the shortened muscles is just as important for this as strengthening the retaining muscles. To support this work, it would be helpful to find some sports activities to improve general endurance levels.

Stretching exercises

With stretching exercises, you are aiming to make all the body's muscles capable of stretching normally and thus to achieve optimum mobility in all the joints. In the hunched posture, the shortening of certain muscle groups occurs over time, causing restriction of movement. Targeted stretching exercises work against this and make the muscles long and flexible again. Flexible muscles make it easier to maintain an upright posture. At the same time, they work better and are more robust from the point of view of injury.

Flexible muscles work better

Stretching postures

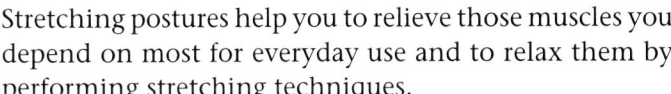 6:00

Stretching postures help you to relieve those muscles you depend on most for everyday use and to relax them by performing stretching techniques.

You should be loose and relaxed for these postures. They should feel pleasant and you should feel no pain at all. Hold each position for at least two to three minutes at first, and increase this gradually.

Stretching posture 1

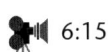 6:15

This first stretching posture is mainly suitable for people who frequently have to stand for long periods of time. Start by lying on your back on a flat mat and place a small cushion or a rolled-up towel under your lower back so

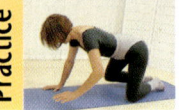
that the lumbar vertebrae are arched and the ribcage raised. Extend your neck and pull your shoulders down toward the lower back. Stretch your arms over your head,

Relief stretching posture after a long period of standing

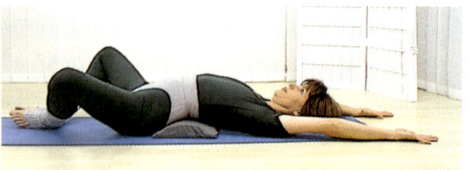

continuing the line of your body, hands flat. If you are unable to lay your arms flat on the mat you may spread them wider.

In this position, pull your feet toward your body. Place the soles of your feet together, facing one another, and allow your knees to drop outward.

6:45 ▶️📹

Stretching posture 2
If you frequently have to sit for long periods, this second stretching posture will help you to relax your muscles. It is similar to the first stretching posture apart from the position of the legs. Instead of bending the legs upward, you stretch them out on the mat and spread them apart as wide as possible.

7:00 ▶️📹

Stretching posture 3
This third stretching posture complements the first two in that it stretches the lateral trunk muscles. Again, you

Stretching posture to extend the lateral trunk muscles

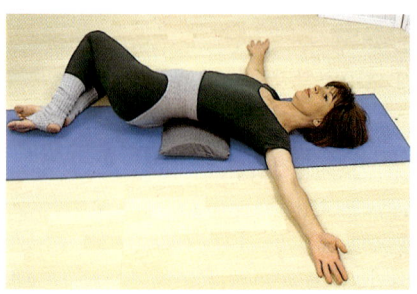

start by lying on your back. This time your arms are stretched out at an angle of 90° to the trunk, the hands flat and turned upward. Both legs are bent upward and the feet are flat on the mat. The knees are then moved to the right from this position, but only while your left arm and shoulder are still on the mat. You should hold this position for two minutes before changing sides.

Top ten stretching exercises for the whole body

7:25

Please follow these instructions carefully when performing the stretching exercises

Go into your selected stretching posture slowly. (By doing this you avoid excessive strain and even injury to your muscles.) You are stretching correctly if you feel a distinct sensation of stretching, but no pain. Do not "flex" or "pull" during the exercise, since this increases the tension in the muscles and you will not achieve the correct stretching effect. Hold the postures for 20–30 seconds and then slowly come out of them. You will then feel a pleasant sensation in your muscles. You will feel the stretching sensation more with some of the exercises described than with others. This means that the shortening in the muscles used is more pronounced and repeated exercising is required. With other muscle groups, which have not been so severely shortened, the exercises are more of a preventative measure.

You should feel the stretching, but as a pleasant sensation

1. The leg and foot muscles

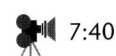 7:40

Stand facing a wall, and about one pace away from it. Lean forward and support yourself against the wall with your forearms. With both feet pointing forward, move one leg forward as if taking a step. Now straighten the rear leg and press the heel into the mat until you feel a stretching sensation in the rear calf. Keep the pelvis parallel to the wall during this exercise, and do not twist it. Raise the ribcage.

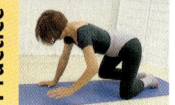
- Hold for 20–30 seconds
- Repeat three times for each leg

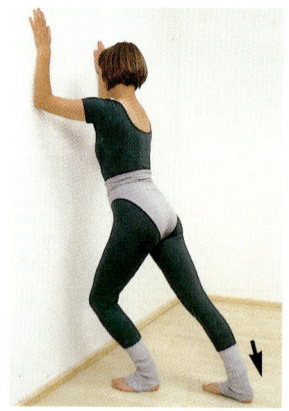

8:05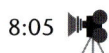

Press the rear heel into the ground

2. The inner thigh muscles

Stretch the muscles of the inner thigh while lying on your back. Place a rolled-up towel under the lumbar region so that you are lying comfortably. Pull your shoulder blades down toward the lower back and extend the neck.

Now bend both your legs, keeping your feet on the floor. Place the soles of the feet together and allow your

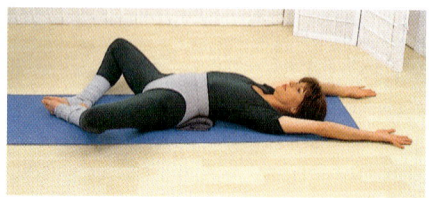

Let the knees fall outward

knees to fall slowly outward. The stretching effect can be increased if you actively press both knees down toward the mat.

- Hold for 20–30 seconds
- Repeat three times altogether

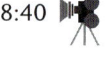

8:40

3. The hip muscles

The basic position for this exercise is kneeling on one knee. Where necessary, support the knee with a cushion or a towel. Place the other knee at a right angle; the first knee remains on the mat. You may support yourself with your hands on the raised leg, but keep the ribcage raised. Now, move your weight forward over the raised leg and push your pelvis forward. Keep the pelvis steady and do

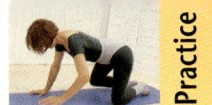

not twist or bend. The stretching effect can be felt in the rear leg, in front of the hip joint. If you do not feel this, raise your knee from the mat a little and stretch the rear leg more.

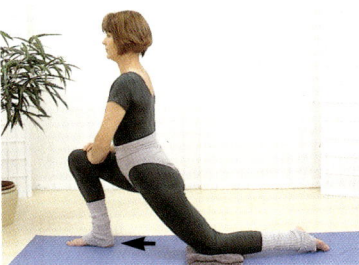

Push your pelvis forward

- Hold for 20–30 seconds
- Repeat three times for each leg

4. The buttock muscles

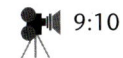 9:10

The basic position for this exercise is on all fours. Bend the elbows slightly, tilt the pelvis slightly and raise the ribcage so that the back is straight. Extend the neck in a straight line with the vertebral column.

Now pull one leg in closer to the body and cross it in front of the other leg so that both knees are in a line. Now push the rear leg back until you feel the stretch effect in your front leg. Both knees remain on the mat

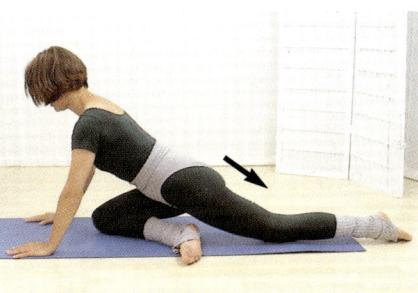

Push the extended leg backward

throughout the stretch. Keep your pelvis steady and do not turn it to either side.

- Hold for 20–30 seconds
- Repeat three times for each leg

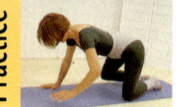

9:45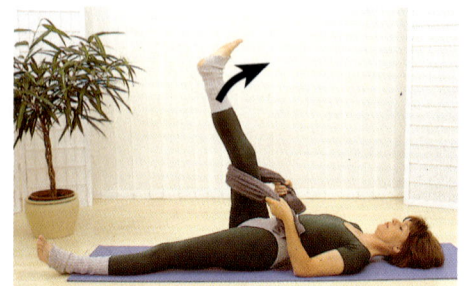

5. The muscles at the back of the thigh

Start by lying on your back. Support the lumbar region with a rolled-up towel. Place another towel under the right thigh and hold one end with each hand. Rest the upper arms on the mat, pull the shoulders down toward the lower back and extend the neck.

Stretch the leg up toward the ceiling

Now bend your right hip by pulling the towel toward you with both hands and keeping the knee bent, until you reach an angle of 90 degrees.

Then stretch the calf upward, straightening the leg toward the ceiling, so that you feel the stretch effect at the back of the thigh. You do not need to straighten the leg completely. You can increase the stretching effect by pointing your toe toward your nose.

- Hold for 20–30 seconds
- Repeat three times for each leg

10:10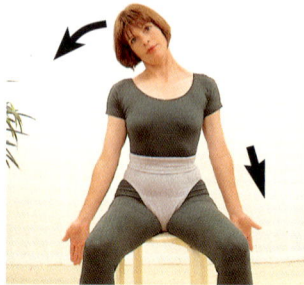

6. The lateral neck muscles

Pull the left hand downward

It is important that exercises are pleasant for the neck muscles too. Dizziness, headaches and other unpleasant sensations may be a sign of incorrect movements or too much strain when stretching.

Stretching exercises for the lateral neck muscles are carried

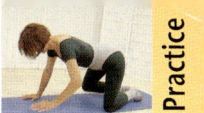
out standing or sitting. Let your arms hang down by your sides, turning slightly outward. Now bend your head to the right, without turning it. Keep the ribcage raised throughout. Push your hands toward the mat until you feel the left lateral neck muscles stretching.

- Hold for 20–30 seconds
- Repeat three times altogether

7. The muscles at the back of the neck

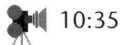 10:35

Sitting or standing, let your arms hang by your sides, turning slightly outward. Extend your neck. Now bend your head to the right. While it is still bent, turn it to face left and bend it

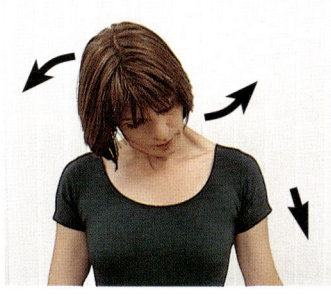

Turn the bent head slightly to the other side

slightly forward. Pull your left hand toward the mat, without touching your body. You will feel the stretching sensation in the left-hand back-of-the-neck muscles. Then change sides.

- Hold for 20–30 seconds on each side
- Repeat three times altogether for each side

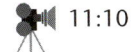 11:10

8. Shoulder and chest muscles

The shoulder and chest muscles – and particularly the main pectoral muscle (musculus pectoralis major) – pull the arms and shoulders forward when they are shortened. When this happens it prevents upright posture. The different groups of these muscles are stretched in three different ways.

Upper shoulder and chest muscles:
Lye on your back. Place a rolled-up towel under the lumbar region. Pull your bent legs toward the body and place your feet on the mat, slightly more than hip-width apart. Place your arms alongside but away from the body,

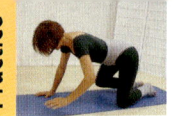

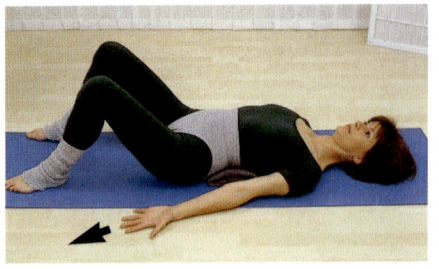

Press the
arms into
the mat, near
the body ...

turn out slightly.
Pull your shoulders
toward your lower
body, keep your
ribcage raised and
neck extended.
Spread your fingers,
extend your arms
and press them
into the mat.

- Hold for 20–30 seconds
- Repeat three times altogether

Middle shoulder and chest muscles:

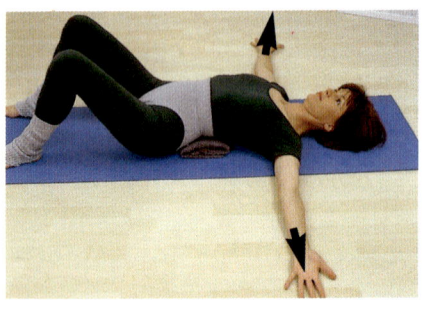

... stretched
out at right
angles ...

In the same start-
ing position, stretch
your arms sideways
and outward, at
right angles to your
body. Now stretch
and spread your
fingers, extend your
arms as much as
possible and push
them into the mat.

- Hold for 20–30 seconds
- Repeat three times altogether

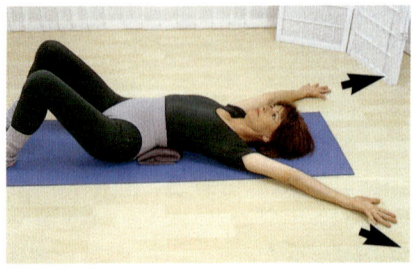

... stretching
over the head
in a V-shape

Lower shoulder and
chest muscles:
Finally, stretch out
your arms above
your head to make
a V-shape. Keep the
ribcage raised and
the neck extended.
Stretch and spread
your fingers and

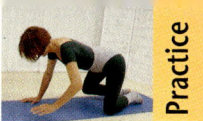

arms and press them into the mat. If your arms do not reach the floor, place a cushion under them and press this down. If this position is painful, try spreading your arms out further away from your head.

- Hold for 20–30 seconds
- Repeat three times altogether

9. The stomach muscles

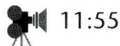 11:55

Carry out this exercise lying on your back. Place a rolled-up towel underneath the lumbar region. Stretch the legs

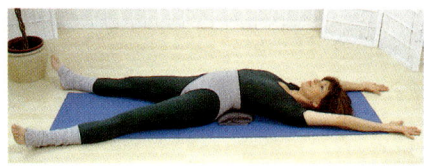

Breathe in deeply so that the stomach rises

and spread them out, then stretch the arms out above the head, extending the line of the body. Pull your shoulder blades down toward your lower back. In this position, breathe deeply and deliberately into your stomach so that the stomach rises when you breathe in and falls when you breathe out.

Breathe in and out slowly and evenly ten times, without holding your breath.

10. Finger and hand muscles

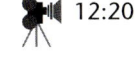 12:20

Standing upright, position yourself about one pace away from, and facing, a wall. Place your hands against the wall at shoulder height and about shoulder-width apart, with outspread fingers. Now, with straight arms, press the wrist joints against the wall.

Take care to keep the ribcage raised and the shoulders down. To heighten the stretching effect, try to raise your

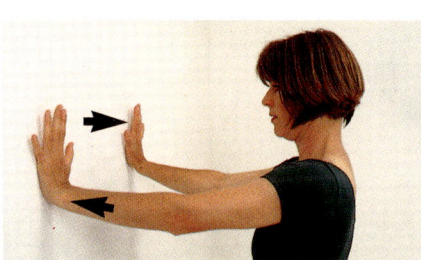

Press the wrists against the wall

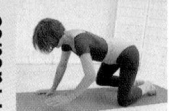

fingers and palms slightly away from the wall, but keep the wrists on the wall at the same time.

- Hold for 20–30 seconds
- Repeat three times altogether

Strengthening exercises

Strengthening exercises make it possible for the muscles to carry the weight of the body, to move or to slow down against the force of gravity more easily and for longer periods. The muscles that are meant to keep the body in an upright position are often too weak for this work because of the hunched posture. They can be toned up using the following exercises. Although one muscle group is targeted in each of them, the whole body will benefit from all of the exercises.

Please follow these instructions carefully when performing the strengthening exercises

Regular exercises, correctly executed

Do your strengthening exercises as regularly as possible – every other day if you can – after the stretching program. After the stretching exercises, the blood supply to the muscles is at its best, and the conditions are excellent for strengthening them.

For each exercise, first adopt the initial position and try to carry out the exercises as exactly as possible, as this is how the "right" muscles are targeted.

Don't forget to breathe!

Try to breathe normally during the exercises. To make this easier, you might count to ten loudly and slowly to start with, because it is difficult to hold your breath while you are speaking. This will also help you to time the exercises correctly.

Maximum hold is maintained for ten seconds and then slowly released. The relevant muscle group should have 20–30 seconds' rest between repetitions. Either allow yourself a short rest or carry out the exercise on the other side of the body in the meantime. Repeat each exercise three times.

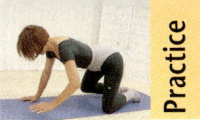
When you begin the strengthening exercises, start with "Program 1: Beginners". If you feel this is not strenuous enough, switch to "Program 2: Intermediate." "Program 3: Advanced" is for more experienced practitioners. Each program can be intensified by increasing the number of repetitions.

The exercises in each of the programs complement each other. Therefore it's best to work your way through the whole program as much as you can.

Program 1: Beginners

🎥◀ 12:40

1. The back muscles

🎥◀ 12:55

1a: On all fours

The initial position is on all fours, with knees and hands on the mat. Place your hands vertically below the shoulders with your fingers pointing slightly outward and the elbows slightly bent. Place your knees a little more than hip-width apart with your feet pointing to each other. Tilt your pelvis slightly forward, raise your ribcage and extend your neck so that your back is straight.

First steady yourself in this position, then raise one arm sideways, at right angles and hold it at body height,

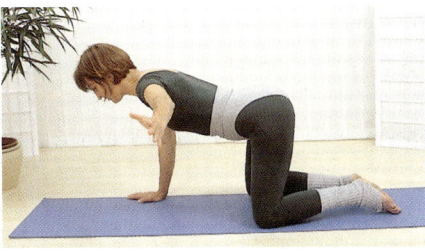

Stretch one arm out at right angles ...

parallel to the floor. Hold this position while counting to ten slowly, then change to the other arm.

- Hold for ten seconds on each side
- Repeat three times altogether

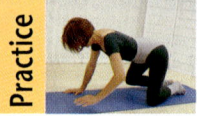
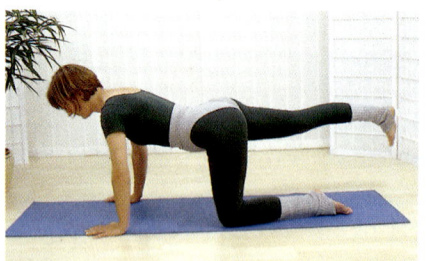

**... then
stretch one
leg backward**

Next, still on all fours, stretch one leg out behind you and hold it at body height. Turn it slightly outward, turning the kneecap slightly outward too. Hold it in this position and slowly count to ten, then change to the other leg. Take care that your pelvis and trunk remain steady during this exercise and do not tend to move sideways.

- Hold for ten seconds on each side
- Repeat three times altogether

13:45    **1b: Lying on your stomach**

Lie down on your stomach on something soft, with legs spread out and the knees turned slightly outward. Place the arms to either side of the body, turning slightly

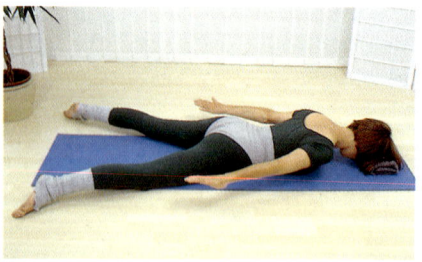

**Make small
circling
movements
with your arms**

outward, with the palms toward the mat. Rest your forehead on a folded towel.

In this starting position, press your breastbone against the mat, extend your neck and pull your shoulder blades down toward the lower back. Now raise your arms and rotate them in small circling movements.

- Continue for ten seconds
- Repeat three times altogether

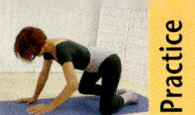

1c: Sitting upright

Sit with an upright body posture on the front half of a chair or stool. With your hands above shoulder level, hold the two ends of a towel. Straighten your arms and raise the towel above your head, then bend slightly forward from the hips, keeping your back straight. Pull the ends of the towel outward and count slowly to ten.

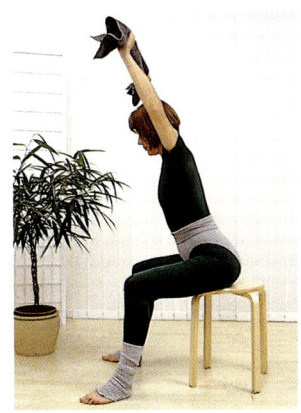

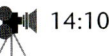 14:10

Pull the ends of the towel

- Hold for ten seconds
- Repeat three times altogether

2. Lateral trunk and hip muscles

Lying on your side

14:30

Start by lying on your side. Place your lower arm under your head and bend the lower leg at the knee, keeping it straight at the hip. Support yourself with your upper arm in front of your body and keep the upper leg straight.

Now lift the upper leg sideways, turning the kneecap

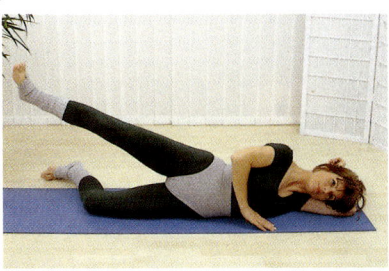

Extend the upper leg, raise and hold

and toes slightly outward. Count slowly to ten. Do not allow the pelvis to slip backward during this exercise. Try to hold the trunk steady and straight. Then change sides.

- Hold for ten seconds on each side
- Repeat three times altogether

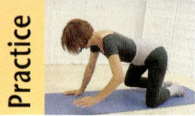

14:55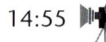

3. Stomach muscles

3a: Sitting upright

Sit upright on the front half of a chair or stool. Place your arms at your sides, and turn then slightly outward. Keep your trunk upright and steady yourself in this position.

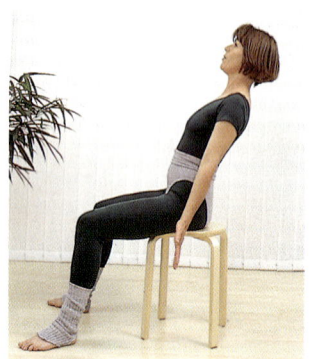

While leaning back, make small movements backward and forward with the trunk

Now bend your upright trunk slightly backward. When doing this, do not form a hollow back: move only your hip joint. In this position, leaning back, make tiny backward and forward movements with your upper body. Count slowly to ten before returning to the initial position.

• Hold for ten seconds
• Repeat three times altogether

3b: On all fours

The initial position for this exercise is on all fours. Place the hands vertically below the shoulders with the elbows slightly bent.

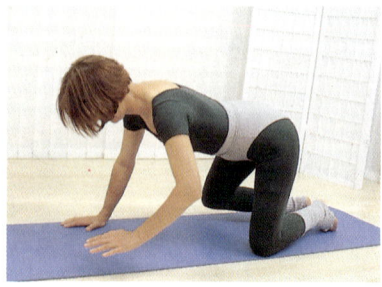

"Trot" on the spot

Place the knees a little more than hip-width apart with the pelvis tilted slightly forward. Extend the neck and pull your shoulder blades down toward the lower back. Steady yourself in this position.

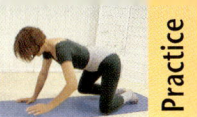

Now raise one hand at a time and the opposite knee at the same time, alternating in small steps. "Trot" like this steadily on the spot.

- Continue for ten seconds
- Repeat three times altogether

Program 2: Intermediate

 15:50

Back muscles

16:05

1a: On all fours

The initial position is on all fours. Place your hands vertically below your shoulders with your fingers pointing slightly outward and elbows slightly bent. Your knees should be a little more than hip-width apart with the feet turned slightly inward. Tilt your pelvis slightly forward, raise the ribcage and extend the neck, so that the back is straight. Steady yourself in this position.

Raise one arm alongside the head, in an extension of the bodyline, the thumb pointing toward the ceiling, and extend the arm at body height, parallel to the floor.

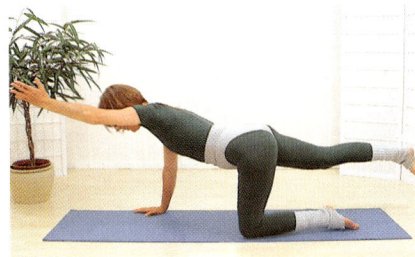

First extend one arm, then the opposite leg

Now lift the opposite leg and stretch it back, holding it at body height. Move it slightly outward and turn it slightly out. Hold while counting slowly to ten and then change sides.

- Hold for ten seconds on each side
- Repeat three times altogether

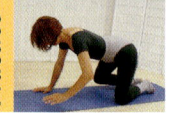

16:40

1b: Stomach position

Lie on your stomach on a soft mat, your legs slightly apart and knees turned slightly outward. Place the arms on the mat at right angles to the body, with the thumbs upward. Rest your forehead on a folded towel.

In this initial position, press your breastbone against the mat, extend your neck and pull your shoulder blades

Make small circling movements with the outstretched arms

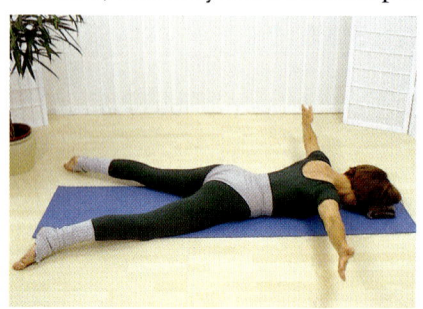

down toward the lower back. Now raise your outstretched arms and rotate them in small circles. Take care not to hold your breath.

- Hold for ten seconds
- Repeat three times altogether

17:05

1c: Sitting upright

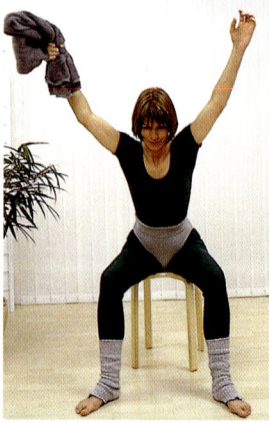

Swing the towel like a lasso

Sit, feet flat, with an upright body posture on the front half of a chair or stool seat. With one hand hold the end of a towel.

Now, keeping your back straight, bend slightly forward through your hip joint. At the same time, keep your arms outstretched above your head and swing the towel in the air in small circular movements like a lasso.

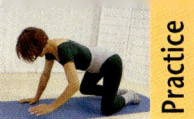

- Continue for ten seconds with each hand
- Repeat three times altogether

2. Lateral trunk and hip muscles

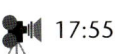 17:20

Lying on your side

Start by lying on your side. Place the lower arm under the head and bend the lower leg at the knee but keep straight at the hip. Stretch the upper arm over your head. Extend you upper leg.

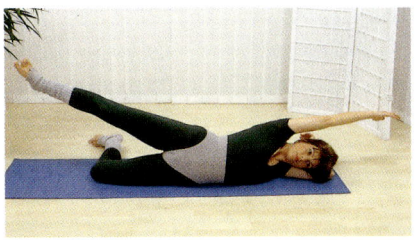

Raise the upper leg while the arm is outstretched

Now lift the upper leg sideways, turning the kneecap and toes slightly outward. Count slowly to ten. Do not allow the pelvis to slip backward during this exercise. Try to keep the trunk steady and straight while holding the position. Repeat three times and then change sides.

- Hold for ten seconds
- Repeat three times altogether

3. Stomach muscles

17:55

3a: Sitting upright

Sit upright on the front half of a chair or stool. Stretch your arms above your head in a continuation of your bodyline. Hold the upper body steady and upright.

Now lean your upright trunk slightly backward. When doing this, do not form a hollow

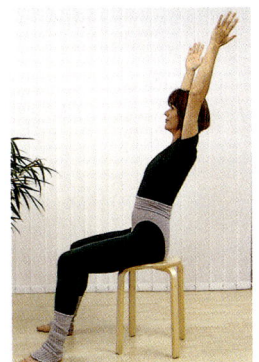

Make small chopping movements with the outstretched arms

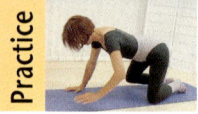
back: the movement is only made at your hip joint. In this leaning-back position, make tiny chopping movements with your arms from the shoulder joints. Count slowly to ten before returning to the initial position.

- Hold for ten seconds
- Repeat three times altogether

18:30

3b: On all fours

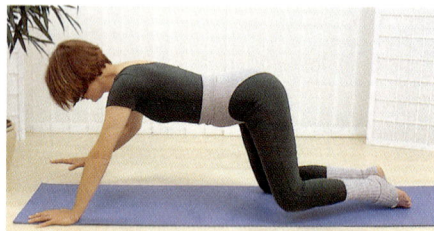

"Trot" with your arms stretched out slightly in front of you

Go on to all fours. This time do not place the hands vertically below the shoulders, but a short distance beyond the trunk, the elbows slightly bent. The knees should be just over hip-width apart. Extend the neck and pull your shoulder blades down toward the lower back. Steady yourself in this position.

Now raise one hand at a time and the opposite knee at the same time, alternating in small steps. "Trot" like this steadily on the spot.

- Continue for ten seconds
- Repeat three times altogether

18:55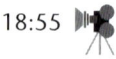

Program 3: Advanced

19:05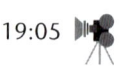

1. Back muscles

1a: On all fours
The initial position is on all fours. Place your hands vertically below your shoulders with the fingers pointing slightly outward and the elbows slightly bent. Place your

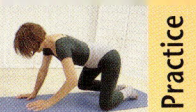
knees a little more than hip-width apart with the feet turned slightly inward. Tilt the pelvis slightly forward, raise the ribcage and extend the neck, so that the back is straight. Steady yourself in this position.

Raise one arm and the opposite leg at body height in an extension of the bodyline and parallel to the floor. Point the thumb toward the ceiling, and stretch the leg

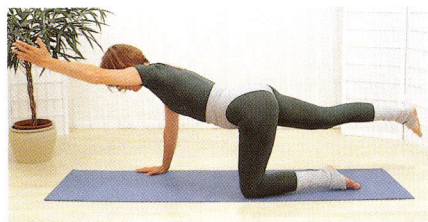

Stretch the arm and leg out at the same time

slightly outward turning it out a little. Hold while counting slowly to ten and then change sides.

- Hold on each side for ten seconds
- Repeat three times altogether

1b: Lying on your stomach

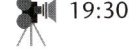 19:30

Lie down on your stomach on something soft, with legs spread out and the knees turned slightly outward. Place the arms close to the head, continuing the bodyline, turning slightly outward, with the thumbs toward the ceiling. Rest your forehead on a folded towel.

Press your breastbone against the mat, extend your neck

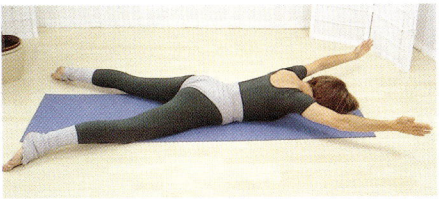

Make small circling movements with your arms outstretched over your head

and pull your shoulder blades down toward the lower back. Now raise your arms and rotate them in small circles.

- Continue for ten seconds
- Repeat three times altogether

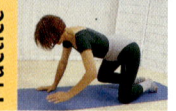

19:55

1c: Sitting upright

Sit with an upright body posture on the front half of a chair or stool. With your hands extended above shoulder level, hold the two ends of a towel. Bend slightly forward from the hips, keeping your back straight. Holding the towel with both hands, stretch it out over your head. Now alternatively bend the arms then straighten them. Keep pulling the ends of the towel outward.

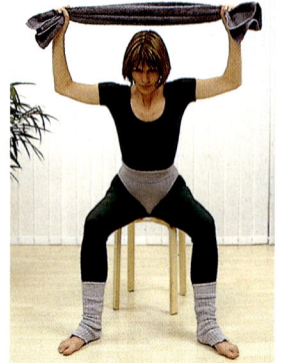

Bend and stretch both arms together

- Continue for ten seconds
- Repeat three times altogether

20:15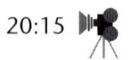

2. Lateral trunk and hip muscles

Lying on your side

You should carry out this exercise in the so-called "supported side position". This means you are in the side position, supported by your elbow and forearm. Bend the lower leg at the knee but keep it straight at the hip. Place the upper arm alongside your body. The upper leg is stretched out. The pelvis is tilted, the ribcage is raised and the neck extended.

Now lift the pelvis from the floor, at the same time pressing down with your arm and the lower leg. The knee remains on the floor. Extend the upper leg slightly

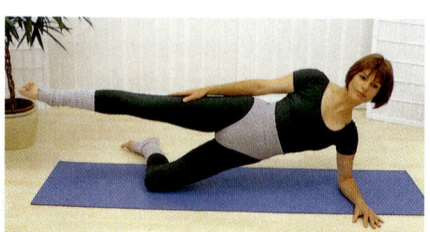

With support on one side, extend the upper leg and hold

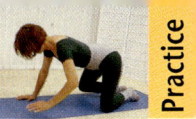

sideways. Turn the kneecap slightly outward. Do not allow the pelvis to bend at the hips or slip back or forward during this exercise. Keep the trunk steady and straight. Hold the position while you count slowly to ten then change sides.

- Hold for ten seconds on each side
- Repeat three times altogether

3. Stomach muscles

20:45

3a: Sitting upright

Sit upright on the edge of a table. You should be at a level where your feet are still flat on the floor. Stretch your arms above your head in a continuation of your bodyline. Hold the trunk upright and steady yourself in this position.

Now lean your trunk slightly backward. When doing this, do not form a hollow back: the movement is only in your hip joint. Raise your legs a little, one after the other, and, with your trunk steady, pull them up a little alternately, like riding a bicycle. Count slowly to ten before returning to the initial position.

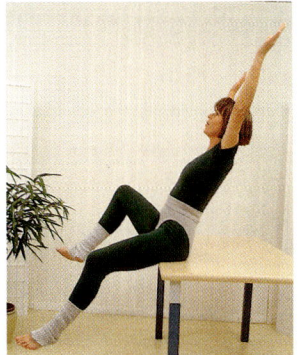

Make "cycling" movements with the legs

- Hold for ten seconds
- Repeat three times altogether

3b: On all fours

21:10

The initial position is on all fours. However, place the hands a short distance in front of the trunk with the elbows slightly bent. Position the knees a little more than hip-width apart. Extend the neck and pull your shoulder blades down toward the lower back. Steady yourself in this position.

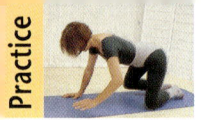

Now raise one knee a little from the floor so that you are standing on tiptoe. In this position, raise one hand at a time and the opposite knee simultaneously, alternating them in small steps. "Trot" on the spot.

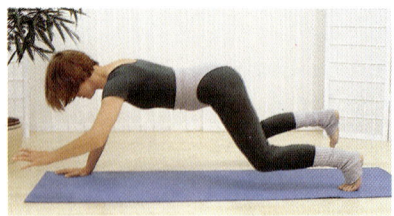

Trot on your hands and the tips of your toes

- Continue for ten seconds
- Repeat three times altogether

Activities that are kind to the back

The following sports and activities complement the strengthening exercises and endurance training. We have deliberately listed those that are kind to the back and that have a compensatory effect after routine overloading of various muscle groups. With regular practice they will improve your physical endurance and promote muscle coordination. On the other hand, other types of sports activities – such as tennis and squash – place an asymmetrical load on the vertebral column.

Note
Activities that are kind to the back and restore physical balance are most effective if you practise them regularly and do not overtire yourself.

Walking and hiking

Walking and hiking provide the ideal physical compensation, especially for people with sedentary occupations. The best pace for walking is at about two paces a second (see page 44). You can be even kinder to your back by making sure you have good footwear. It should fit well i.e. be neither too big nor too small, nor too narrow or broad. The shoes should

Two steps a second

to keep your back fit

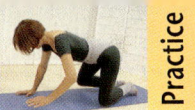

be firmly fitted to the feet and should support the arch with a suitable insole. The soles must be flexible and be able to follow the rolling movement of the foot. The heel should be two centimeters high at most and should, where possible, have a buffer action.

Walking and hiking in brief:
Endurance training: very good
Strengthening: very little
Risk of injury: low
Important: good footwear

Jogging

Jogging is ideal for endurance training if you bear in mind the following points: deliberately choose a slow speed. You will know you have reached the right speed if you can still have a normal conversation without getting breathless. At every step, set each foot down heel first and roll it forward. As when walking, the point of the foot turns slightly out if you do this. The ribcage is raised and the shoulders hang loosely to either side, with the arms slightly bent and actively following the running movement, with open hands. Make sure you have good footwear. A soft, absorbent surface is ideal for minimum loading of the joints.

Jog slowly and use your whole foot

Jogging in brief:
Endurance training: very good
Strengthening: good
Risk of injury: exists
Important: good footwear, see walking

Swimming

For the back, the indisputable advantage of swimming is that, in the water, the body is free of the burden of gravity. This means greater scope for activity under less weight for the vertebral column and the muscles. The breaststroke offers the most suitable training for an upright posture. In order not to constantly over-extend the cervical vertebrae and cause damaging overloads, the head should be under water while executing the stroke. One way of avoiding this is to swim on your back. Although this is often recommended unreservedly it is important to remember that, to achieve the optimum alignment of the vertebral column, your head must also be in the water. If you lift your head out of the water, your body hunches again.

High activity but low weight-load

With the crawl, and even more so the butterfly stroke, the everyday hunched posture is encouraged even more by the arm movements and muscle activity: these strokes are not, therefore, recommended.

Swimming in brief:
Endurance training: very good
Strengthening: very good
Risk of injury: low
Important: think of the right position for the cervical vertebrae

Cycling

Toning the leg muscles

Cycling provides excellent training for the leg muscles, especially if you sit or stand a lot during the day. The traditional "Dutch," or "sit-up-and-beg," cycle is ideal for an upright posture. This allows you to cycle with a straight back with the trunk leaning forward slightly. The broad handlebars of this type of bicycle also promote a raised ribcage. On the other hand, the narrow dropped

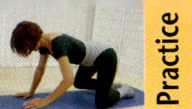

handlebars of racing cycles mean that the shoulders are pulled forward and the back rounded. However, if you prefer a racing cycle for speed, you should keep the stages short and always do compensatory stretching exercises afterwards (see page 57).

Cycling in brief:
Endurance training: very good
Strengthening: very good
Risk of injury: low
Important: think of the right size for your body and adjusting the cycle

Riding

Contrary to popular opinion, riding is an activity that *is* good for the back. After a certain learning period, it is possible to ride in an upright position, with the pelvis tilted and the ribcage raised. As far as the back is concerned, however, the "English" style of riding is unsuitable due to the use of the pelvis to control direction, a practice that involves loading the stomach and buttocks. Such movements, which are often used in classical dressage, are very damaging to the vertebral column. On the other hand, riding for pleasure, even with a light saddle, may be recommended for toning the muscles of the torso. Since, in addition to other groups of muscles, the thigh muscles are mainly involved, we recommend you practice stretching postures and exercises after riding (see page 55).

Upright posture

Riding in brief:
Endurance training: good
Strengthening: good
Risk of injury: exists
Important: remember to do stretching work on the thighs afterwards

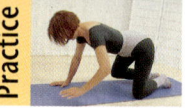

Dancing

Ballroom dancing for posture

The upright posture required for dancing supports regular posture training during the course of everyday activities. The type of dancing that is most suitable for endurance training for the back is mainly ballroom. The backward bends of the spine in more energetic styles of dancing are, on the other hand, more damaging and should be avoided for the sake of a healthy back.

> **Dancing in brief:**
> Endurance training: good
> Strengthening: good
> Risk of injury: low
> Important: comfortable shoes are good for the back.

Relaxation and relief for the back

Relaxation

Relaxation is a central component of any training for the back. Back pain is in most cases attributable to hardened and overloaded muscles. Some simple relaxation techniques will help you to gradually reduce this "permanent stress" in your muscles.

There are many methods of relaxation

Depending on personal preference, you can choose your relaxation methods from a wide spectrum: ranging from "Autogenic Training," via yoga to the different methods of meditation. However, all of these very varied techniques have one thing in common: the effectiveness of each stands and falls on correct practice.

One very effective and easily learnt method is known as "Progressive Muscle Relaxation". This technique was described by an American, Dr. Jacobson, at the beginning of the century and means the same as "Relaxation Through Tension". Although it sounds like a contradiction, it works!

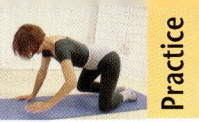
Awareness exercise

If you clench your hand very firmly into a fist, you will find that the forearm tenses at the same time. It can even be painful, depending on how much tension you apply. You can really feel it when you tense your muscles. Now release the muscles. You no longer feel the tension. The muscles of the forearm have relaxed.

If you understand this difference between tension and release, you will also be able to learn the Progressive Muscle Relaxation technique. This involves tensing and then releasing all the major muscle groups in your body one after the other. There are many guides to this technique. If you are interested, we recommend the Sehbuch video *Balance – Stress-Free and Relaxed in Minutes*. (See the Further Reading section on page 89 for more information on this subject.)

However, there is also a range of other relevant techniques you could easily learn with the right guidance. Evening classes offer courses on the subject of relaxation. You simply need to look at the program and choose the techniques and courses that appeal to you. If all this seems too expensive and too complicated and you would rather do something more spontaneous for yourself, then a regular visit to the sauna, possibly followed by a massage, a warm bath or walks in the country can be wonderful ways of finding a sense of relaxation. The most important thing is that you take some time out for yourself and fulfil your need for relaxation.

Relaxation takes time

Relief postures

The following relief postures will help you to ameliorate acute tension in your back and provide support, and

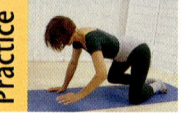

therefore relief, for your vertebral column during long uninterrupted periods sitting down or standing.

Raising your feet while lying down

This position, which is used mainly for pain relief with lumbago or a slipped disk, involves raising the feet. The individual lies on the floor with legs raised to an angle of 90 degrees and supported by a cushion. Generally, another substantial pillow supports the head. Seen from one side, it is easy to see that the person concerned is lying in a hunched position.

To achieve a straight posture, the pillow should only be thin and, if the pain allows, a folded towel should be

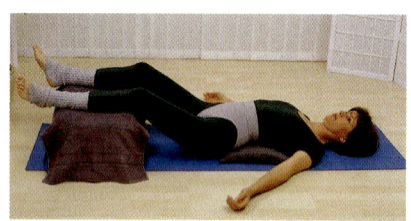

Raising your legs while using a lumbar cushion

placed under the lumbar region. Instead of the excessively high leg support, another roll under the knees is often enough to reduce the pain.

Stretching postures are also useful for relief of strain in the vertebral column (see page 55).

Note

If you suffer from sudden severe back pain, let your doctor know immediately. Raising your feet, as described here, will only help to make acute pain more bearable and is no replacement for the correct treatment of, for example, a slipped disk.

Relief postures: sitting

There are various ways of providing short-term support, and therefore relief, for the vertebral column if you sit for long periods. However, you should still maintain an upright posture throughout. Tilt your pelvis, raise the

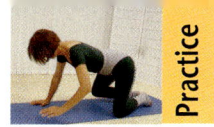

ribcage and extend the neck. Try the following positions in any order.

Sit leaning back in an upholstered chair:

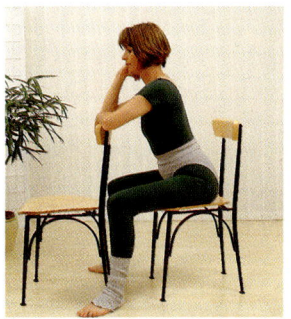

Keeping your back straight, support your head on your hands

- still sitting, lean your upright trunk forward from the hips and use your hands to support your head with extended neck
- place your hands on your head and stretch your trunk back over the chair back, keeping your trunk straight
- while sitting, rest your arms to either side on the chair armrests
- rest both your hands on your thighs

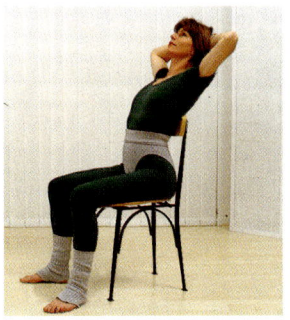

Keeping your back straight, stretch your trunk back

- sit the wrong way round on a chair and support yourself with your forearms on the chair back
- sit sideways on a chair and lean against it sideways.

Relief postures: standing

You can also take the strain off your vertebral column in certain positions when standing. You should still take care to maintain an upright posture throughout. Try out the following positions in any order.

- Lean with your back against a wall and support one foot against the wall.
- Support yourself by "half sitting" on the edge of a table or desk.
- Support your upper body with your arms, for example against a wall or on a table.
- Holding the top of a doorframe with both hands, bend your knees so that your arms take your body

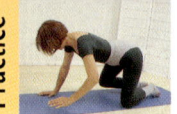
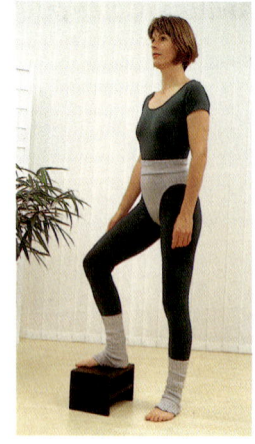

Place one
foot at a
higher level

weight and the vertebral
column is extended.
• Place one foot slightly higher
than the other.

Ways to relieve stress

Relief remedies support your
vertebral column by encouraging
its natural S-shape. They take the
strain from the muscles that are
normally responsible for this and
help to prevent strain when you
have to sit for extended periods
of time.

Lumbar support

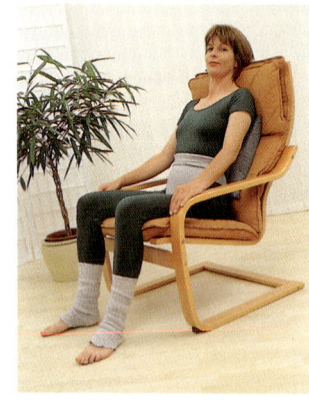

A lumbar
cushion
supports and
takes the
strain from the
vertebral
column

Lumbar support cushions
come in varying sizes and
thicknesses. When you lean
back in a seat, they support
the lumbar vertebrae in
their natural alignment.
They also make it easier to
raise the ribcage. Lumbar
cushions can be used at any
time and anywhere – with
office chairs, armchairs, and
in car seats – especially
when you have to sit for
long periods of time. A lumbar cushion can also be used
to support the vertebral column when you are lying on
your back (see page 51). It is a good idea to fold a hand
towel and use it to find the right size and thickness for a
lumbar cushion.

Hint
If no lumbar cushions are available (for example, on a

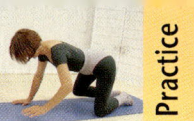

train or at the cinema), you could use an item of clothing or a bag to support your back.

Wedge cushion

A wedge cushion is a wedge-shaped cushion which is higher at the back than the front. When used on a chair seat, it supports the pelvic tilt forward and downward and thus helps you to maintain an upright posture. It is particularly useful in the workplace when sitting forward – for example, when writing. It can also be used to neutralize the effect of chairs where the seat itself slopes backward.

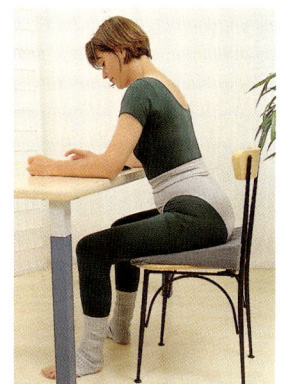

The wedge cushion encourages the pelvic tilt

Home heat-treatment remedies

Warmth has the effect of stimulating the blood supply and it therefore encourages tensed muscles to relax. This is why there are countless simple and effective practical household remedies that can be used to apply warmth to muscle cramps and pain and thus help to alleviate acute back pain.

Warmth promotes muscle relaxation

With hot compresses and packs, it is clear that they should be applied directly to the painful area to soothe the pain. However, back pain may also often be displaced pain, where the cause lies in other muscle groups (see page 29). For problems with bending, it may for example be the stomach or buttock muscles that are responsible. This means that hot compresses will still be soothing, if they are applied to those areas. Neck pains can be helped by hot treatments applied to the inside of the forearm or by a hot footbath. All these methods depend on individual preference, however, and the heat must always be soothing and not unpleasant.

Taking a rest after every heat treatment is not only pleasant, it is also sensible. The rest period may well include stretch postures (see page 55), as these have an additional soothing effect on the vertebral column and back muscles.

Hot-water bottle

A hot-water bottle is the simplest way to apply heat. Simply half-fill with hot water, squeeze out the air and close it. It is best suited for contact with the body's surface when filled like this. Place the hot water bottle on the desired part of the body and leave it there for about 10 minutes.

Moist heat

The effect of a hot-water bottle is enhanced if you place a moist flannel between the skin and the bottle. The water used in this case should be almost boiling. If it is too hot, let the hot-water bottle cool off first.

Moist heat heightens the effect

Heated pad

A heated pad has the same use as a hot-water bottle but is not as effective.

Hot compress

For a hot compress, a hand towel is folded in half – depending on its length – and then rolled into a cone shape and filled with boiling water. The towel should be warm and completely soaked, but not dripping wet. The roll is gradually unrolled from outside in, so that every section of the towel is used.

Hot and highly effective

Cornflower compress

Cornflowers are gathered during haymaking. Little sachets of dried cornflowers can be bought at the chemist's. They can be placed in a dish or a sieve and steam heated. They are then placed on the relevant part of the body and left for as long as they retain their heat.

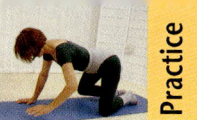

Potato compress

The potato compress makes use of one property of potatoes – their good heat retention. To make up a potato compress, hot potatoes, boiled in their skins, are mashed and wrapped in a cloth. This hot pack is placed on the body and left for as long as it retains its heat.

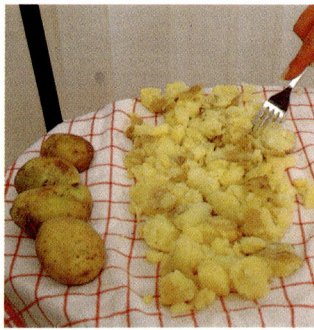

Potatoes have good heat retention

Footbath

A hot footbath can bring relief to back pain and strain in the neck and upper back and in many cases to headaches. Place your feet in a suitable container which you have filled with hot water. The feet should be covered up to the level of the mid-calves. If you have varicose veins you should ask your doctor if a hot footbath is suitable.

Sauna

The beneficial effect of a sauna depends on alternately overheating and cooling the body. This stimulates the metabolism and the blood supply and, as a result, the muscles relax, general mobility improves, heart and circulation are toned, breathing deepens and the immune system is reinforced.

Alternating heating and cooling cycles stimulate the metabolism

Since a visit to a sauna has a marked effect on the heart and circulation, you should take advice from trained sauna staff before using one for the first time. After going to a sauna a period of rest, preferably lying down, is absolutely necessary (see page 50) until your metabolism returns to normal.

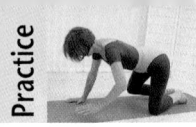

Relaxation
for the body
and relief for
the mind

Warm bath

A warm bath relaxes the body and is beneficial for the mind. The temperature of a warm bath should be between 36–38°C, and various herbal preparations can enhance the pleasant effect. The effects are comparable with those of a sauna. The heart rate and circulation are relatively rapid, so that if there is any doubt you should consult a doctor first about whether a bath is advisable. After a bath, a period of rest is recommended, preferably lying down (see page 50).

About the authors

Dr. Bernard C. Kolster is a medical doctor and physio-therapist. He has long been concerned with themes involving physical medicine, the rehabilitation process after severe illnesses and operations, oriental medicine, and natural remedies. Over the last few years, Dr. Kolster has published several books and films in these areas which are read both by specialists and the general public. Astrid Frank is a trained remedial therapist/physiotherapist and Bruegger therapist. She has, for many years, been active in the training and advanced training of remedial therapists/physiotherapists and regularly runs posture and back training courses in-house for various organisations as well as training instructors in this area. As an author, she has already been involved in several publications in the field of back training, physiotherapy, and pain therapy.

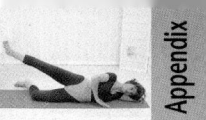

Appendix

Further reading

Gray, Timothy J. Back Works. Book Partners Inc, Washingon, USA 1993.

Oliver, Jean. Back in Line. Butterworth-Heinemann, Oxford 1999.

Sherwood, Paul. The Back and Beyond. Arrow Books Limited, London 1992. Sutcliffe, Jenny. Solving Back Problems: Simple Techniques for a Pain-free Back. Marshall Pulishing 1999.

Wilson, Andrew. Are You Sitting Comfortably? Optima, Ebury Press, London 1994.

Other videos in this series

Kolster, Bernard C.: Partner Massage. Cologne, 1999

Kolster, Bernard C.: Reflexology. Cologne, 1999

Kolster, Bernard C.: Shiatsu. Cologne, 1999

Kolster, Bernard C.; Cernaj, Ingeborg: Balance. Cologne, 1999

Appendix

Index

Arthritis of the joints 32

Back pain 20
- psychosomatic 36
Bath, warm 88
Bed 50
Bending 45

Carrying 49
Chair position 53
Cog wheel model 13
Compress, hot 86
Cornflower compress 86
Cycling 78

Dancing 80
Defective posture 21
Disks 9

Everyday environment 53
Exercise ball 54

Footbath 87

Getting up 39

Heat, compress 86
Heat, moist 86
Hollow back 22
Home remedies 85
Hot water bottle 86
Hump back 21

Jogging 77

Lifting 47
Lumbago 30
Lumbar cushion 84
Lying down 50
Lying face down 52
Lying on your back 51
Lying on your side 51

Mashed potato compress 87
Muscles 11

Osteoporosis 34

Pillow 51
Posture 12
- hunched 13
- upright 15
Posture training 39
Progressive Muscle Relaxation 80
Psychotherapy 37

Raising your feet 82
Relaxation 80
Relief postures 81
Relief remedies 84
Riding 79

Sauna 87
Sciatica 33
Scoliosis 23
Sitting 40
Sleep 50
Slipped disk 32, 82
Spinal cord 8
Splay foot 17
Standing 44
Stomach muscles 24
Strain 26
Strengthening exercises 64
- back muscles 65, 69, 72
- lateral trunk and hip muscles 67, 71, 74
- stomach muscles 68, 69, 71
Stretch postures 55
Stretching exercises 57
Swimming 78

Upper back syndrome 28

Vertebra 8
Vertebral column 7

Walking 44, 76
Wear and tear of the joints 32
Wear and tear of the vertebral column 3
Wedge cushion 85
Work table 54